ETHNOGRAPHY IN NURSING RESEARCH

MNR
Methods in Nursing Research

SERIES EDITOR
Pamela Brink, R.N., Ph.D.

The purpose of the **Methods in Nursing Research** series is to provide basic references to designs, methods, and sampling procedures not readily available in other formats. Each book is designed to be a complete reference to any single topic.

Books in This Series . . .

Ethnography in Nursing Research
Janice M. Roper
Jill Shapira

Forthcoming:

Hermeneutic Phenomenological Research
Marlene Z. Cohen
Richard H. Steeves
David L. Kahn

ETHNOGRAPHY IN NURSING RESEARCH

Janice M. Roper
Jill Shapira

MNR
Methods in Nursing Research

Sage Publications, Inc.
International Educational and Professional Publisher
Thousand Oaks ■ London ■ New Delhi

For information:

Sage Publications, Inc.
2455 Teller Road
Thousand Oaks, California 91320
E-mail: order@sagepub.com

Sage Publications Ltd.
6 Bonhill Street
London EC2A 4PU
United Kingdom

Sage Publications India Pvt. Ltd.
M-32 Market
Greater Kailash I
New Delhi 110 048 India

Printed in the United States of America

Library of Congress Cataloging-in-Publication Data

Roper, Janice M.
  Ethnography in nursing research / by Janice M. Roper,
Jill Shapira.
    p. cm.— (Methods in nursing research; v. 1)
  Includes bibliographical references and index.
  ISBN 0-7619-0873-0 (cloth: acid-free paper)
  ISBN 0-7619-0874-9 (pbk.: acid-free paper)
  1. Nursing—Research—Methodology.   2. Ethnology.
3. Qualitative research.   I. Shapira, Jill.   II. Title.   III. Series.
  RT81.5 .R66 2000
  610.73'072—dc21   99-050407

This book is printed on acid-free paper.

00   01   02   03   04   10   9   8   7   6   5   4   3   2   1

Acquiring Editor:	C. Deborah Laughton
Editorial Assistant:	Eileen Carr
Production Editor:	Sanford Robinson
Editorial Assistant:	Victoria Cheng
Designer/Typesetter:	Janelle LeMaster
Indexer:	Molly Hall
Cover Designer:	Candice Harman

CONTENTS

Series Editor's Foreword   vi

Preface   viii

1. Overview of Ethnography   1

2. Ethnography as Method   11

3. Headwork and Footwork: What You Do Before
   Writing the Proposal   29

4. Writing the Research Proposal   39

5. Getting Your Foot in the Door   55

6. Now Go Do It!   65

7. What to Do With All the Data   91

8. Ethical Responsibilities   113

9. Annotated Bibliography   125

References   135

Author Index   143

Subject Index   146

About the Authors   149

SERIES EDITOR'S FOREWORD

This is the first of a series of books on research methods in nursing. The purpose of the series is to provide basic references to designs, methods, and sampling procedures not readily available in other formats. The books are designed to be a complete reference to any single topic and can be used without further explanation or help from a tutor.

This first text, *Ethnography in Nursing Research*, is an excellent example of what the series is expected to accomplish. Many educators and researchers have a very confused notion about ethnography, a research design developed by anthropologists for anthropologists. The design is based upon participant observation as the primary data collection method supported and enhanced by other data collection methods such as interviewing, available data, artifacts and so on. In fact, ethnography is the original "mixed method" and as such has the strength of longitudinal research and triangulation of methods.

Some nurse researchers assume that they are doing an *ethnography* if they are using the interviewing style described by James P. Spradley, when in fact they are using a single data collection method developed for a specific kind of ethnography. Others believe that if they are using a data analysis technique used by anthropologists, that they are doing *ethnography*. Neither of these beliefs are true, as this text shows.

Janice Roper and Jill Shapira, both trained anthropologists, have produced an excellent work on doing ethnography in a hospital setting. Drawing on their combined considerable experience, they explain what an ethnography is and what it is not, how it has evolved in nursing, and how it is used by nurses in a hospital setting. The book can stand alone as a guide and a reference to ethnography as a research method. I believe you will find it a very useful, as well as highly readable, book.

Pamela J. Brink, R.N., Ph.D.

PREFACE

This book is written for nurses who have little or no experience conducting ethnographic studies. We write this book from our own experiences as researchers and clinicians. Many of the examples provided are from our own background. JR is a researcher who has conducted qualitative research as an investigator in a large metropolitan medical center. Specifically, her qualitative work has encompassed an observation study in an admissions area, ethnographic analysis of the use of restraints and seclusion in an intensive care psychiatric unit, and use of combined ethnographic methods and quantitative methods in a study of agitated behaviors in Alzheimer's disease patients and the impact of these behaviors on caregivers (with JS). In addition, she teaches research to nursing staff at the medical center, with an emphasis on qualitative research methods. Last, she is currently a member of one of the human subjects subcommittees' institutional review boards (IRBs) in the center.

The research experience of JS includes a longitudinal study of spouses acting as caregivers that focused on a qualitative analysis of open-ended interviews, an ethnographic study in the emergency room, coinvestigation with JR on the agitation study, and currently a focused ethnography on the phenomenon of agitation in one surgical intensive care unit as part of her doctoral study in anthropology, where she has recently been advanced to candidacy.

Our research efforts have been developed from clinical questions that puzzled us. The projects focused on distinct problems, and we formulated research questions before conducting the studies. These research experiences were confined to medical center settings and were considered problems relevant to patient care and supported by nursing services. Finally, we both worked within our own nursing "culture" to gain insights into common occurrences and taken-for-granted everyday events.

This book is about ethnographic methods, that style of research introduced to us by Dr. Pamela Brink. Ethnography is a process of learning about people by learning from them. The concept of ethnography developed within the tradition of anthropology, as lone anthropologists went into "the field" to study "exotic" people. Ethnographers use three methods to describe cultural entities and groups of people. By observing what is happening, participating in activities and then asking the "natives" about what is seen and what is being done (interviewing), and examining existing documents, the ethnographer gains a deep understanding of the practices and beliefs of the group.

We assume that you have no or minimal experience with the methodology of ethnography. We also assume that you have had a beginning-level introduction to research, either through academic courses or by participating in the conduct of someone else's study. Thus, we have not defined usual research terms except as they apply to ethnographic research. We also assume that you will have a mentor or advisor to assist you with learning the conduct of the ethnographic methods and analysis of your ethnographic data. Ethnography is a methodology that requires experience. It cannot be learned adequately from books and journals.

We believe that the concepts and descriptions of methods described in this book apply to research in all settings, whether in a familiar place with one's own cultural group or among a group of people with different beliefs and perspectives of the world. The book is meant to be read consecutively, but each chapter has enough detail to be read alone. Chapters 2, 6, 7, and 8 are about the actual conduct of ethnographic research, the analysis and interpretation of the data from your fieldwork, and ethical issues in ethnographic research. Chapters 3, 4, and 5 describe the processes related to putting your ideas into writing and gaining access to the "field." So depending on your level of knowledge in relation to these broad subject areas, you might find it beneficial to read selected chapters according to your needs.

The overview of ethnography presented in Chapter 1 includes a discussion of how traditional classical ethnographic concepts become more focused in many studies. In Chapter 2, we present an overview of ethnographic methods. (For more detail about the methods, the reader is referred to Chapter 6.) In Chapter 3, we outline important issues to consider and tasks to perform before writing the research proposal, including formulating an appropriate research question, negotiating with the potential field site, and deciding on the need for funding. Concrete suggestions for writing the research proposal and special considerations of ethnographic studies are discussed in Chapter 4. In Chapter 5, we delineate steps in obtaining formal institutional approval. We have placed in Chapter 6 a detailed description of how to collect information in ethnographic studies. Specific techniques of sampling people and events, observation, and interviewing informants are provided. General methods used to analyze participant observation data are included in Chapter 7. Chapter 8 discusses ethical considerations related to the role of being an ethnographer and the reflexivity associated with this research process. In Chapter 9, an annotated bibliography, we have abstracted information from ethnographic studies conducted by nurses. Many of these are also referenced in the text.

We view ethnography as a very personal experience, one that requires time, commitment, and dedication. In this book, we have presented an overview of the ethnographic process and methods that we hope will help you. We wish you success in your endeavors to learn from others.

1

OVERVIEW OF ETHNOGRAPHY

> . . . to grasp the native's point of view, his relation to life, to realize
> *his* vision of *his* world.
>
> Bronislaw Malinowski,
> *Argonauts of the Western Pacific*
> (1922, p. 25; emphasis in original)

Ethnography is a research process of learning *about* people by learning *from* them. This approach is used by investigators to understand
and describe why a group of people do what they do. The principal
methods used by ethnographers are participant observation, interviewing, and examination of available documents. Through ethnographic
participant observation, the researcher systematically observes and personally participates in activities of group members to experience the
flow and patterns of community life. Formal and informal interviewing
are also part of ethnography and allow the investigator to discover the
salience or meaning that observed patterns of behavior have for group
members. In addition, the ethnographer reviews supplementary sources
of information, including written reports, visual records, and historical
accounts, to obtain a broad perspective of the people, setting, and research issues. The researcher's observations, feelings, and understand-

ings gleaned from participant observation, interviewing, and additional sources, are documented in field notes, which are then analyzed to reveal answers to the questions asked by the research project. The result of this written description and analysis is called ethnography; thus, ethnography is both a process and a product. This approach allows the investigator to experience events with group members while maintaining the professional distance necessary to conduct research. This blend of "knowing" from both an insider's perspective and an outsider's analysis allows deep and rich insights about the behaviors and beliefs of individuals as they navigate their social world.

The purpose of this book is to describe principles and methods of ethnography used by researchers, specifically nurse-researchers, who examine issues related to health and illness. The aim of this chapter is to provide an overview of this ethnographic perspective. We first identify concepts and characteristics intrinsic to traditional or classical ethnographies. We then situate and discuss medical ethnographies within this traditional framework. We end the chapter with a description of the more focused ethnographies conducted by nurses and other clinically oriented ethnographers.

CHARACTERISTICS OF ETHNOGRAPHY

Ethnography is a description of the patterns of behavior of individuals and groups of people within a particular culture (Agar, 1986; Bernard, 1994). The concept of ethnography—going out into "the field" and describing a group of "exotic" people—evolved within the framework of cultural anthropology. The British anthropologist Bronislaw Malinowski is generally viewed as the originator of intensive field research, although his systematic methodology was influenced by W. H. R. Rivers, a physician-anthropologist-psychologist who did fieldwork in the Torres Straits in 1898 (Stocking, 1983). Malinowski lived with the people of the New Guinea Trobriand Islands for a total of 2 years and experienced "constantly the daily life of the natives . . . , while accidental, dramatic occurrences, deaths, quarrels, village brawls, public and ceremonial events, could not escape . . . notice" (Malinowski, 1922, p. xvi). Malinowski (1922) believed that because they were so "interwoven, the totality of all social, cultural and psychological aspects of the community" should be considered (p. xvi). In addition to his vivid descriptions, Malinowski analyzed the motives and feelings of the people whose behaviors he observed. The principles and methods used by these early anthropologists form the foundation for current ethnographic studies and are highlighted below.

The ideology of *culture* is fundamental to the discipline of anthropology, but it is a term hard to define. There are two main conceptualizations of culture: behavioral/materialist and cognitive (Fetterman, 1989; Spradley & McCurdy, 1972). From the behavioral/materialist perspective, culture is observed through a group's patterns of behavior and customs, what they produce, and their way of life (Harris, 1968). According to the cognitive formulation, culture consists of the ideas, beliefs, and knowledge that are used by a group of people as they live their lives. The rules of a specific culture are learned, and they tell members how to behave appropriately: what to eat, what to wear, how to speak, and what to believe about the world. By applying these two concepts of culture, ethnographers determine what people know and believe and what they do.

Traditionally, anthropologists conducting ethnography live with small groups of people (100-500 members) whose ways of life are greatly different from their own. To discover their behavior patterns and knowledge systems, they focus on the exotic and the unusual in descriptions of these cultures (Chagnon, 1992; Malinowski, 1922; Mead, 1968; Turner, 1967). The same techniques are also used to understand the cultural rules of individuals in urban settings: Spradley's (1970) ethnography of homeless men in one city of the United States and the description of an Italian neighborhood by Whyte (1955) are two examples. Regardless of the setting of these ethnographies, the general questions guiding the studies are the same: What is it like to be a member of the particular culture? What are the rules guiding social behavior?

To understand a culture in its totality, the ethnographer strives for a *holistic perspective* that captures the breadth of activities, knowledge, and beliefs of the group under study. In addition, the information that is learned is *contextualized* by being placed within a larger perspective. Everything the investigator observes—the events, behaviors, and relationships within a cultural group—is analyzed in conjunction with the meanings it holds for individuals, as well as historical influences upon the process. To comprehend the culture of a group different from one's own with this degree of depth requires *intensive face-to-face contact* over an *extended period of time.* Ethnographers become enmeshed in the lifeways (Leininger, 1985) of the people by studying real-life situations as they occur in their *natural setting.*

To collect these data, the ethnographer uses *participant observation,* an "umbrella of activity" that encompasses a variety of techniques (Schatzman & Strauss, 1973, p. 14). By observing what is happening, participating in activities, and then asking members about what was seen and done, the investigator gains a deep understanding of the practices and beliefs of the group. Through the process of participant observation, the ethnographer initially discovers the insider's view of the world, the *emic perspective.* The goal is to identify peoples' categories of meanings and the way "the natives define things" (Pelto & Pelto, 1978, p. 62). In addition, the investigator brings the outsider's framework, the *etic perspective,* to the field of study. This is the view used as the ethnographer observes events and then tries to make sense of what is seen by identifying patterns of behaviors. There is an attempt to be "objective" by providing definitions and scientific explanations drawn from the investigator's cultural background. Ethnographers use both perspectives by participating in experiences and then stepping back and analyzing the data collected. There is also the recognition that ethnography is "neither subjective nor objective" (Agar, 1986, p. 19) but results from the interpretations made by the ethnographer. This *reflexive* aspect assumes that the researcher is a part of the world being studied and is influenced by the experiences and relationships that he or she encounters (Boyle, 1994). According to Werner and Schoepfle (1987), "This combination of insider/outsider provides deeper insights than are possible by the native alone or an ethnographer alone. The two views, side by side, produce a 'third dimension' that rounds out the ethnographic picture" (p. 63).

In summary, classical ethnographic studies depict human behavior, beliefs, and values within a cross-cultural perspective. The aim is to develop scientific generalizations about different societies by comparing political, economic, kinship, and religious aspects of the social framework that organizes behavior (Leininger, 1970). Descriptions of illness and health practices appear as components of these social systems; examples include the relationship of religious beliefs and disease causation and healing rituals conducted for specific illnesses or processes of birth and death (Chagnon, 1992; Lévi-Strauss, 1963; Turner, 1967). However, information obtained about processes of disease and illness in traditional cultural ethnographies is generally fragmentary and unsystematic (Landy, 1977, p. 12). A subfield of medical ethnography evolved within cultural anthropology to specifically examine the cultural components of medical beliefs and practices.

MEDICAL ETHNOGRAPHIES

The term *medical anthropology* was first used by Scotch (1963) to describe the discrete field of study within anthropology that focuses on the human response to health and illness that is embedded within cultural systems (Landy, 1977, p. 1; Wellin, 1978, p. 23). Today, anthropologists, sociologists, nurses, physicians, social workers, occupational therapists, and other social scientists conduct medical ethnographies. We provide but a few examples from this rich and diverse body of literature that reflect (a) the relationship between cultural beliefs and health behaviors of community members and practitioners and (b) the ability to study the "cultures" of specific illnesses and health processes.

Medical ethnographers conducting community studies describe in great depth the relationship between cultural beliefs and health behaviors of community members. Arthur Rubel, an anthropologist, lived among Mexican American immigrants of a South Texas town in the late 1950s. In his ethnography, Rubel (1966) first provided an account of the lifeways of these Americans of Mexican descent and then related this cultural background to the processes used to cope with health problems. He also explored the cultural significance of anxiety and disaffection among members of this community. Rubel vividly described the behaviors and meanings behind health practices. He also situated the community within a historical perspective and thus acknowledged both microlevel and macro-level processes related to cultural behavior. Although the purpose of this research was to produce a Chicano account of health issues, Rubel also considered the perspective of the physicians and some of their problems in providing care for members of this Mexican American community and illuminated the relationship between two different cultural groups. Another researcher who did a community medical ethnography was Margarita Kay (1977), a nurse anthropologist who also worked within a Mexican American barrio. She asked the following question: "What do we need to know about people in order to tailor health care to them?" Kay first situated health practices of the people within their general cultural system by participating in community activities and interviewing women from several generations. In addition, she identified general features of illnesses common in the community. She then used an etic perspective to compare and contrast Mexican American views of illness with the biomedical model of disease. Like Rubel, Kay grounded her findings and recommendations within a firm cultural context that strengthened her conclusions.

Some medical ethnographers investigate specific illnesses or expected developmental processes to discover common beliefs and practices of patients or practitioners or both. Sue Estroff (1981) conducted fieldwork in the 1970s with a chronically mentally ill population in her own city. Rather than studying the culture of a group, she examined the culture of an illness. Although she generally considered the lives and perspectives of patients in this ethnography, she also presented the treatment team's perspective of working with these community patients. She represented individual, social, and political aspects of the complex problem of mental illness within the United States. The interplay between micro-level and macro-level components of the system enriched her discoveries and comments. Similarly, Dona Lee Davis (1992) explored the meaning of menopause in a Newfoundland fishing village. She identified the impact of sociocultural factors in shaping women's experiences of middle age, specifically the social expectation of enduring hardship and the shared value of an egalitarian ethic within this community.

In sum, these medical ethnographies resemble traditional or classical ethnographies. There is a major emphasis by the researchers on discovering how cultural understandings inform health beliefs and practices. Intensive personal contact between ethnographer and participants occurs where people live or work. The interplay between micro-level and macro-level processes situates and contextualizes the findings within a broad perspective and provides a holistic portrait of specific health phenomena within the larger social world.

Clinically oriented ethnographers employ the general approach of medical ethnography but concentrate their emphasis upon the local worlds and practices of individuals in relation to specific issues of health and illness (Kleinman, 1992, p. 130). Topics of inquiry are selected before data collection begins; participant observation activities are confined to specific places, times, and events; and interviews are structured around the subject of study. Although the participants may come from different cultural backgrounds, they share the experience of a particular illness (Morse & Field, 1995, pp. 154-155). To study distinct and delineated health concepts within a contextual perspective, nurses and other clinically oriented ethnographers conduct focused inquiries.

FOCUSED ETHNOGRAPHIES

Most nursing ethnographies today focus on a distinct problem within a specific context among a small group of people. This type of ethnography is labeled *focused ethnography* (Morse, 1987, pp. 17-18), *miniethnography* (Leininger, 1985, p. 35), or *microethnography* (Werner & Schoepfle, 1987). These studies answer questions that are formulated before going into the field, and the knowledge learned is expected to be useful and have practical application for health care professionals (Muecke, 1994, p. 187). Because the intent is to concentrate efforts on very specific questions, the research can be accomplished within a shorter time than traditional ethnographies. Focused ethnographies share with classical ethnographies a commitment to conducting intensive participant observation activities within the naturalistic setting, asking questions to learn what is happening, and using other available sources of information to gain as complete an understanding as possible of people, places, and events of interest. We provide examples of focused ethnographies by nurse-researchers studying (a) specific health practices among diverse cultural groups, (b) specific community settings as sites of supportive activities, and (c) the practice of nursing as a cultural phenomenon.

Pioneer nurse anthropologists used focused ethnographic methods to discover how people from various cultures integrated health beliefs and practices into their lives. For example, Pamela Brink (1982) described the practices of traditional birth attendants among the Annang of Nigeria and compared them with the practices of American and Nigerian hospital-based obstetrical teams. In this study, Brink discovered the effectiveness of the majority of strategies used by the rural attendants and made suggestions to encourage the use of clean techniques during the birthing process. In another focused ethnography, Janice Morse (1984) described and compared traditional beliefs and customs regarding infant feeding in the Fijian and Fijian-Indian cultures. This study revealed that hospital staff were generally unaware of the prevailing cultural practices that influenced infant feeding in these societies. Finally, Juliene Lipson and her colleagues (Lipson & Omidian, 1997; Lipson, Hosseini, Kabir, Omidian, & Edmonston, 1995) examined the difficulties faced by Afghan refugees in the United States. Ethnographic data were collected for more than 10 years and included intensive interviewing and visiting in homes of several families, participating in social occasions, driving individuals to scheduled appointments, and acting as advocates with health or social service providers. The authors discovered, among other findings, that inadequate or misunderstood information contributed to problems in obtaining health care services for many members of this community. Thus, through their research endeavors, these nurse ethnographers helped nurses realize that cultural groups have health practices that fit their own particular way of life (Leininger, 1970, p. 47). Discovering salient beliefs and behaviors of patients permits nurses to deliver culturally competent and ethical care (Tripp-Reimer, Brink, & Saunders, 1984).

Focused ethnographies are also conducted in urban areas among specific subcultural groups of the larger society. Karen Kauffman (1995) studied a senior center in an inner-city ghetto and its elderly African American members in the early 1990s. She posed the question: "How do elders survive in the midst of 'drug warfare' in an inner-city community known for its dangerous streets and public spaces?" Kauffman participated in community activities for 3 years, including spending 3 to 4 days each week at the senior center, attending grassroots organizational business meetings, and going to evening and social events. She discovered that the general fear of being victimized was lessened by participation in the senior center. She situated her findings within a larger context of violence in urban America and then described how actual and potential violence affected the social health of individuals. Gary Carr (1996) also examined a specific subset of the American population. In his ethnography of an HIV hotel, he considered the meanings of the hotel as a supportive community for marginalized individuals who shared the experiences of HIV, meanings of drug use for hotel residents, and meanings of working in this specific site for nurses. Understanding the meanings that members of this subcultural group assign to their experiences may help nurses plan and provide needed care.

In addition to the health practices of diverse cultural and subcultural groups, focused ethnographic methods are used to study the practice of nursing as a cultural phenomenon. Sally Hutchinson (1984) conceptualized a newborn intensive care unit (NICU) as a cultural system and explored the interactions of nurses to discover what it is like to be a nurse in this setting. Similarly, Germain (1979) portrayed patients and staff of an oncology unit as members of a highly specific community with unique patterns of behavior and described and analyzed societal, institutional, and individual factors affecting their interactions. Street (1992) was also interested in the ways nurses' practice and critically examined the nursing profession within historical, biomedical, and feminist frameworks. These ethnographic examples view nursing as a subculture with unique beliefs and practices within the general health care system. Their descriptions illuminate the nursing culture and become part of nursing history (Germain, 1993, p. 266).

The focused ethnographies discussed in the above paragraphs retain the characteristics of traditional ethnographic inquiries. Both describe individuals and groups within a holistic perspective and aim to uncover cultural beliefs and practices that generate observed behavior (Brink, 1976, p. 2; Leininger, 1970, p. 2; Osborne, 1969, p. 11). Comparing variables in different cultural groups or health care settings allows for a better understanding of the complexities of common situations; theories may then be developed and tested in other situations. In addition, careful attention is given to the "participant's" or "patient's" emic view of the world. Etic insight into meanings behind actions—why people do what they do or believe as they do—is a principal outcome of ethnographic studies.

We discuss the specific methodology of ethnography in this book. The essential principles of ethnographic analyses include the concept of culture and a commitment to obtaining a holistic perspective of the world-view and behavioral patterns of individuals and groups and phenomena of interest to nurses. Ethnographies are designed to collect three types of information, which are then interwoven to allow broad and deep understandings of people and how they interact in their social world. In the next chapter, we present an overview of the principal methods of ethnography—participant observation, interviewing, and examination of available documents—and describe their characteristic features.

2

ETHNOGRAPHY AS METHOD

Anthropology is a field that celebrates complexity and ambiguity in a world looking for simplicity and clarity.

M. H. Agar, *Show It, Don't Tell It* (1996, p. 3)

QUALITATIVE FRAMEWORK FOR ETHNOGRAPHIC RESEARCH

Ethnography is one type of a qualitative research design. Qualitative research, in general, aims to consider the holistic context in which meaning is assigned to experiences. The conduct of all qualitative research is an interactive process of inquiry between the investigators and the participants.

Several approaches or styles fall under the general heading of qualitative research. Three of these are ethnography, phenomenology, and grounded theory research (Lowenberg, 1993). Though all three approaches may use similar data collection strategies of participant observation and interviews, they differ in their overall goals, the types of

TABLE 2.1   Overview of Qualitative Methods

Type	Research Question	Focus
Ethnography	What are the beliefs and practices of veterans living in the shelter	Describes experiences within the cultural context
Phenomenology	What is the lived experience of electroshock therapy?	Captures the essence of experiences
Grounded theory	What are the processes by which adolescents with cancer achieve sexuality?	Generates concepts leading to theory development

questions they ask, and the specific techniques they use to answer the questions (Table 2.1). What they share is a commitment to understanding everyday life experience from the participants' point of view.

Ethnographic studies describe various perspectives of the participants within an interactive social context (Lowenberg, 1993). Ethnography itself includes a number of techniques. In traditional anthropology, ethnography is synonymous with fieldwork. Anthropologists have used a variety of ethnographic techniques to understand and learn about non-Western cultures. In nursing, these methods are used to study aspects of nursing and health care. The practice of nursing is a rich environment for ethnographic research (Dreher & Hayes, 1993; Street, 1992).

When ethnography is the methodology of the investigation, researchers themselves become the instruments for data collection (Burgess, 1984b; Morse, 1989; Ragucci, 1972). The influence of the investigator on the outcome of the study is of concern to ethnographic researchers and to others who question the objectivity of the method. Does the investigator change the interactions, responses, and behaviors of the participants? How does the investigator separate his or her "self" from the data? If it is possible to use the self as a data collection instrument—how is it learned? We discuss these issues related to role definition of the ethnographer within the context of participant observation in this chapter. The aim of the chapter is to present an overview of ethnographic methods and how they are used by nurses in research.

ETHNOGRAPHIC METHODS

Ethnography involves three possible data collection strategies: participant observation, formal and informal interviews, and examination of available related documents—a natural triangulation of investigative approaches on the same phenomenon.

The process of ethnography is inductive. Although the researcher conducting a focused ethnography is guided by general topics of interest and even specific questions to be answered, there are no or minimal preconceived notions about the *outcomes* of the research. The questions formulated before the actual fieldwork begins guide the research and are subject to change as the study progresses (Morse, 1991).

PARTICIPANT OBSERVATION

Although the approaches of grounded theory and phenomenology use participant observation to augment information collected in interviews, an ethnographic approach makes participant observation its central strategy. Becker and Geer (1984) defined participant observation as gathering data by participating in the daily life of a group or organization (p. 239). Spradley (1980) viewed ethnographic fieldwork not as "studying people" but as "learning from people" in the sense of discovering what the world is like to them (p. 3). Thus, the focus becomes an active involvement in social events as they occur in their natural setting.

Dimensions of Ethnographic Participant Observation

Germain (1979), in a study of nurses within a hospital unit, listed seven dimensions that the researcher must explore to achieve subjective adequacy within ethnographic participant observation. First is the amount of *time* required for the study. As an ethnographer, you must spend enough time in the setting to learn about the people, behaviors, and events and to be accepted as a member of that group. You must have enough time to witness and participate in activities and to follow though on pertinent issues to their conclusion. There seems to be no general rule about the amount of time to spend, but there are reports of fieldwork that lasted years and of fieldwork that lasted only a few months or weeks. *You* have to be the judge of whether you are spending enough time in the setting. At least three factors will influence this judgment. First, your own personal situation may place limits on the amount of time you can spend being an ethnographic participant observer. Also, the organization or setting where your research is being conducted may limit the amount of time they will allow you in their institution as an ethnographic participant observer. Finally, the research question will influence how much time you spend as an ethnographic participant observer. When you recognize that your research question has been answered and you are getting no new information (referred to as *saturation*), it is time to "leave the field" (Gagliari, 1991).

The second dimension to be explored is *place,* or the location or locations where ethnographic participant observation is to be conducted. The appropriate setting is necessary to answer your research questions. If you want to study rituals in nursing practice, nursing practice must be observed. The location of particular phenomena to be studied must be identified. For example, Fisher and Peterson (1993) were interested in describing attitudes of operating room staff toward elderly patients. To accomplish this aim, they spent 5 months as participant observers in three operating rooms at one inpatient facility and also interviewed physicians and nurses. They concluded that surgeons in particular had negative attitudes toward the elderly that resulted in disregard of the patients' dignity and in performance of procedures that were not done on younger patients. Estroff (1981) wanted to understand the world of psychiatric patients, so she spent 2 years as a participant observer in the Program of Assertive Community Teaching (PACT) for the recovering mentally ill. Carr (1996) studied the developing cultural milieu in a hotel that provided housing for persons with HIV by observing activities in the setting and interviewing staff. When conducting ethnography, you have to go to a place where the population and problems are related to your study topic.

The third dimension to be explored is *social circumstances.* To have a complete picture of the setting and its people, the researcher benefits from attending social events in the setting, as well as formal organizational activities such as meetings and classes. Kauffman (1994) found that trust was built with the participants in her study when she joined them in the social events of the community. In that study, the investigator was young and white, whereas the participants were elderly and black. Participation in social events allowed the researcher to overcome the barriers presented by age and ethnicity and greatly enhanced her understanding of the participants in her study.

The fourth dimension is *language*. If you are studying your own culture and subculture, you may not have trouble with an unfamiliar language. However, conducting ethnography in your own language may cause you to miss relevant communication patterns because of your familiarity and accompanying insensitivity to nuances. On the other hand, lack of knowledge about a language may benefit the study. Field (1989) reported that Iranian emigrant women revealed to her (a non-Iranian) details of their personal lives that were not revealed to the other investigator, a person from Iran. It was speculated that the Iranian women were uncomfortable about sharing this very personal information with someone from their own culture. If you are not fluent in the language of your participants, you may have to engage an interpreter/translator. This has been the case in a number of ethnographic participant observation studies (Kulig, 1988, 1995; Lipson, 1989; Morse, 1984; Muecke, 1992).

Fifth is the dimension of *intimacy*. You will want to become involved in the setting as closely as possible without losing your objectivity. Inherent in the ethnographic participant observer role is the need to become "immersed" in the culture, the event, and the phenomenon (Gans, 1984). Also recognize, however, that the setting and its members may put limitations/restrictions on what you may see. Gender differences may limit your access to certain events. During her work with community psychiatric patients, Estroff (1981) realized that being female was both a hindrance and an advantage. Most of the mentally ill patients in her study were men, many of whom had little contact with women. Her gender allowed her to gain access to the group of patients; however, it later became a disadvantage when the participants made sexual advances to her. There were some activities, therefore, that she simply missed because of her gender and her refusal to respond to the sexual advances.

Sixth is the dimension of *consensus or validation* of data and interpretations of the data. Validation is performed in a number of ways. You can check *your* interpretation with that of participants in the study. For example, after observing the placement of patients in restraints, Roper (Roper & Anderson, 1991), asked these same patients about their experiences: Did they know why they were placed in restraints? Did the restraints help? What were their feelings about restraints? This informa-

TABLE 2.2   Dimensions of Ethnographic Participant Observation

Element	Qualities
Time	Can be weeks, months, or years Influenced by *your* time, your research question, and the setting
Place	Appropriate to answer your research question(s)
Social circumstances	Become part of the ethnographic participant observer process/role Increase knowledge and understanding of phenomena
Language	Ethnography in your native language or in a setting of another language may present barriers to understanding
Intimacy	Becoming involved with group members without losing objectivity
Consensus/validation	The steps taken to ensure your interpretations are accurate
Bias	The worldview that you bring to the field of study; also, others' view of you may create bias

tion from the patients served to validate her observations that patients were not informed about the process, did not understand the purpose of restraints, and were opposed to their use. Further, you can check your observations and interpretations of what you have observed with the participants through informal interviewing. These processes are discussed in detail in Chapter 7.

Finally, you must always be aware of *bias,* which may influence your data collection, interpretation of findings, and description of findings. Bias can work in a number of ways. The obvious, of course, is the worldview that you bring to the setting—your personality, values, belief systems, and knowledge. Less obvious is the bias of the participants toward you. Participants may restrict access to information or even give you wrong information because you are not a member of their group. Germain (1979), while studying clinical nursing on an oncology ward, reported that administration, without explanation, barred her from attending administrative nursing functions such as structured meetings and reports. Thus, she was not able to consider this information when interpreting her findings—a form of bias. To increase the potential for a cooperative relationship with your participants, you need to maintain an open, nonjudgmental attitude and listen attentively to the statements of the group members. Be clear about your role, and explain how you expect to interact with the group and how the information you learn will be used (Table 2.2).

Levels of Participant Observation

Four levels or roles of involvement in participant observation re search are generally recognized: participant, participant-as-observer, observer-as-participant, and observer (Burgess, 1984b; Byerly, 1969). Most ethnographers move back and forth among these levels (Burgess, 1984b; Schwartz & Schwartz, 1955) but spend most of their time being participants-as-observers or observers-as-participants.

The four levels of participant observation are placed on a continuum from most involvement with the participants (participant only) to no involvement with the participants (observer only). Most ethnographic information is collected when the researcher is in the role of participant-as-observer or observer-as-participant. The use of a specific role is driven by the situation. Brink (1982) illustrated the movement between roles in her study of birthing techniques among the Annang of Nigeria. When she viewed a birthing, she was an observer, but immediately after the birth she was more participant-as-observer as she accompanied (and often drove) the new mother and infant to their home.

Similarly, Wing (1990) was able to distinguish very clearly between her data resulting from direct observation and data collected using ethnographic participant observation. Direct observation was conducted as nurses went about their work in their natural environment. This technique enabled the investigator to compare the actual nursing behaviors that she observed with the described accounts from the nurses themselves. Participant observation was a dual role, so information could be learned as the researcher became a participant in the research setting and worked alongside the nurses. When a participant-as-observer, Wing had access to areas that were not available to her as an observer. In the participant-as-observer role, she was more involved in the culture and could see events and actions from an insider's point of view.

We stress that the method of participant observation used in ethnographic research involves a majority of time spent actively participating in the activities of the group members. Thus, ethnographic participant observation combines the modes of participant-as-observer and observer-as-participant. However, there are times when the ethnographer becomes primarily an observer of or primary participant in selected events.

Participant-as-Observer. We have found that the participant-as-observer role increases the likelihood that the researcher will obtain key "insider" information about what it is like to be a member of the cultural group. This role also enables the researcher to validate observations with the participants while observing, interpreting, and recording. The important thing to remember is that participant observation takes time. Your position will evolve from that of stranger to that of someone who is to varying degrees accepted by members. If you are already a member of the group you are studying, such as a nurse in the setting where you work or a nurse in a health care setting where you are not known, you may have a jump on the process. Be prepared, however, to be tested in relation to your participation in the group. Seed (1995) used participant observation to immerse herself in the world of the student nurse. During the early phase of being a participant observer, she identified episodes in which students tested her trustworthiness by seeing if she would report situations where policy was violated or patient care was left undone. The investigator did not breach the confidentiality of the student nurses. By the end of the study, the students no longer questioned her trustworthiness.

In the role of participant-as-observer, the nurse investigator ideally moves between the nursing role and the observation role with fluidity. But these transitions may be problematic. It is tough to be both insider and outsider. The differences in roles may confuse the participants in your study. They may become suspicious of your participant/researcher role changes, Roper (Roper & Anderson, 1991), as a member of the nursing staff but not of the ward she studied, was able to be a participant-as-observer. She participated in ward activities and assisted staff with patients. But the observer role was difficult to achieve and maintain. As an employee of the study site for years, she was recognized as both a participant in patient care and an administrative-type nurse. Staff frequently queried her about changes happening in the hospital. Some staff even tried to get her involved in the work role by asking, "Can't you do something about. . . ?" Or they would monitor their behavior around her, saying things like "I wish you hadn't seen that" or falling silent when she came in the room. Some staff asked the head nurse if she was a "spy" for administration, although no staff shared that opinion with her. These behaviors lessened over time.

Observer-as-Participant. While in this mode, the ethnographer's contact with informants is briefer and more formal. Reduced participation in activities is expected as observations are made. The goal is to collect specific information. Or the setting may not allow a greater degree of participation. Street (1992) and Germain (1979), in their ethnographies, were examples of observers-as-participants. Neither were members of the staff that they studied. These investigators accompanied nursing and other staff as they carried out their nursing activities, but did not directly provide care to patients. Conducting an ethnography using *only* the role of observer-as-participant is problematic. The briefness of the encounters with the culture/subculture means there is less chance for validation of observations with the members and more opportunity for bias to influence interpretation of events, actions, and behaviors. It may also be less satisfying to the researcher because the observer as participant is transient in the environment. The researcher is probably not included in any insider activities (Burgess, 1984b). Nevertheless, some subject matter may lend itself to this strategy of data collection. For example, you may want a contrast or comparative group for specific information related to your overall study and be able to justify obtaining the data in this limited fashion.

Using the combination of participant-as-observer and observer-as-participant roles, the ethnographer has the best opportunity to perceive events and understand meanings. Researchers using these roles can also step back from the situation, interpret their observations, and analyze the event. Although the observer-only and participant-only roles may be used on a limited basis in some parts of your study, the real essence of ethnographic participant observation is the combination of participant and observer roles.

Observer Only. In the observer-only role, the researcher does just that—*observe only,* with no participation in the members' activities. This total outsider role is the most distanced from the "insider" perspective. The advantage of this mode is that observers may be more objective, but much data may be lost because the researcher will not obtain any of the insider information. The observer-only approach is appropriate for only brief periods of time during an ethnographic project.

Pure observation, however, can be very enlightening if done correctly, despite the basic limitations of the method. Schwartz and Schwartz (1955) described the use of the observer or "passive" role in a study of need fulfillment on a ward. Observers recorded the requests of patients and staff response to the requests in order to count the number of requests and responses. Their *observer-only* status gave them the freedom to attend only to what was the focus of the observation; in doing so, however, they missed other events that related directly to the focus (p. 348). If a portion of your ethnography would benefit from collecting observation data only, one way to increase the effectiveness of data collection would be to seek information on where and when it would be best to make the observations in order to "catch" the phenomenon (Street, 1992). For example, Roper (Roper & Anderson, 1991) used the mode of observation only to identify where events took place on the psychiatric ward. During this observation-only period, she learned that events important to her study took place in the hallways.

The epitome of an observation-only study is Rosenhan's (1973) study in which students became pseudopatients in psychiatric facilities to study definitions of normality and abnormality. The presence of these pseudopatients was unknown by clinical staff in the 12 inpatient settings. The pseudopatients ceased demonstrating "psychiatric" symptoms once they were admitted to a ward and became observers. The pseudopatients took notes on their observations of the ward, other patients, and staff. The only way to leave the setting was to convince the staff that they were "normal." Although patients on the wards identified the pseudopatients as impostors, none of the staff made such observations. The pseudopatients were labeled with psychiatric diagnoses, despite their seemingly normal behavior. The method of observer only was appropriate for the research question asked in this study, but would require justification in today's research climate.

Salyer and Stuart (1985) conducted observation-only research of nurse-patient interactions in an intensive care unit (ICU). They labeled the 217 interactions that they observed as "negative" or "positive." There was no validation of the researchers' labels with the staff or patients. This study was not an ethnography, but it demonstrates the limitations of conclusions drawn from observations that have not been validated with the participants. We do not recommend that this approach be used alone.

Participant Only. As participant only, the investigator is intimately involved with the setting, people, and activities under study. We do not feel comfortable with this role, as covert observation is involved (Burgess, 1984b). In addition, research review boards probably would not approve this type of study. One advantage of the participant-only stance is the probability that the investigator will be accepted as one of the members of the group and thus be privy to "insider" information. The disadvantage is that the researcher may lose perspective and objectivity as an insider.

In addition, because the role of observer is covert, the group members are subjects of a study without knowing about it or agreeing to participate—an ethical issue. Last, in participant-only research activities, there is the possibility that the researcher will change the culture/group/organization or will totally "go native," leaving data collection and research behind (Burgess, 1984b). It is Gans's (1984) position that it is almost impossible to be totally immersed in a culture and at the same time observe oneself and others. Diamond (1992) studied nursing assistants in nursing homes using the participant only approach. While conducting the research, he was a paid nursing assistant at the facilities. No one knew that he was conducting a study. Data collection was covert. Nursing assistants, patients, and administrators did not know they were subjects in a study. Though Diamond described in rich detail the practices of nursing assistants, the avoidance of obtaining informed consent is questionable in that his research role was concealed.

Generally, when beginning fieldwork in a totally new environment, the ethnographer moves from an observer position into the position of participant-as-observer or observer-as-participant. If, and when, the role becomes one of participant only, it is time to leave the field or risk abandoning the role of researcher and going "native."

INTERVIEWS

A simple overview of interviewing strategy within ethnography is provided here. More detail is provided in Chapter 6.

Interviews are used to validate observations made during ethnographic participant observation and to provide direction for future observations. They are also used to gather data related to issues that you may not have observed, that you cannot observe (e.g., the participants' thoughts), or that you cannot reliably ascertain by observation (e.g., the participants' feelings). For example, if your subject matter is like that of Khazoyan and Anderson (1994)—Latinas' expectations of their partners during childbirth—you must query your informants.

Interviews may be formal or informal. Informal interviews are not prearranged; they involve asking questions about an event or interaction immediately after it occurs to check participants' perceptions against your own. For example, when you say what you saw and what you think occurred in an event, the participant may agree with what you say and offer more explanation or may contradict your observation and give you new and different insights. Dreher and Hayes (1993) were able to increase the validity of their study by checking their observations of children with the parents and teachers. In other cultures or settings, participants may not be so willing to assist you. They may in fact react with hostility or be upset by your questions and refuse to answer.

Formal interviews involve some planning, such as making up an interview guide covering a list of topics or specific questions that you want to explore with informants. As in informal interviews, questions are open-ended. The interview can be structured in various ways. Spradley (1979) suggested initial global questions followed by more specific descriptive, structural, and contrast questions to focus questioning further. Mac-Donald (1996) used the in-depth interviewing strategies of Spradley (1979) to learn about mothers of children with asthma. On the basis of the initial interview with the mothers, she developed descriptive, structural, and contrast questions for subsequent interviews.

Interviews are often tape recorded for transcription, coding, and interpretation. If, as in many studies (Khazoyan & Anderson, 1994; Kulig, 1998, 1995; Lipson, 1989; Morse, 1984; Muecke, 1992), the interview must be conducted in the participants' native language, you may have to hire a translator unless you are proficient in the language of your participants. For example, Khazoyan and Anderson's (1994) study of a Latina population required translating interview questions into Spanish and then translating responses back into English for coding and interpretation.

Remember that the formal interview must be related to your research question and purpose of your study. It cannot be conducted merely for the sake of curiosity. Most nursing ethnographies are focused. Exploration is conducted around specific phenomena or issues. The data from such interviews are coded for interpretation in relation to the rest of the study and are used to supplement and verify participant observation data.

EXISTING DOCUMENTS

Existing documents that may be pertinent to your research question and the focus of your study include maps, policies, procedures, patient records, results of tests, biographical material, and census figures. They may take a wide variety of forms. Cook and de Mange (1995), studying non-Native American nursing researchers' access to Native American cultures, found it useful to examine historical documents related to distrust of non-Native Americans, sociopolitical structures, and specific problems and needs of the Native American group that they were studying. Magilvy, McMahon, Backman, Roark, and Evenson (1987), in their study of teenagers in a town in Colorado, consulted secondary epidemiological data, both to understand the community and to validate the participant observation and interview findings. Other kinds of documents that might be consulted are medical records, such as records of tests, exams, and related medical procedures. Of course, specific permission is usually required to access these private documents.

Be creative in identifying the documents that will help you with your study completion. Music, videos, and books may also support the needs of your study. When permission is required, be sure to request it in a timely manner.

In sum, we have described three methods used in ethnographic research: participant observation, interviews, and consultation of existing documents. If you use all three, you will be able to triangulate your findings—the subject of the next section.

TRIANGULATION

Denzin (1978) first advocated triangulation as a method to enhance the validity of qualitative research. Triangulation can involve the use of multiple methods of data collection related to your subject matter (as in ethnographic research) or the use of more than one theoretical framework or analysis method. Generally, in ethnographic research, triangulation is achieved through the three methods of participant observation, interviews, and examination of existing documents. For example, if you were studying depression among Vietnam veterans, data could be obtained directly from veterans, using an open-ended interview that would explore what depression meant to veterans. Documentation in these patients' medical records might be the second source of information. A third source might be participant observation data on veterans and their families or veterans and staff. The three forms of data would provide a total picture of depression for the group under study and would serve to validate each other.

Ethnographic nursing research provides many examples of studies that draw on these three data sources to perform triangulation. Field (1983) used participant observation, formal and informal interviewing, and perusal of client records and clinic reports to study four public health nurses' perspectives of nursing. Engebretson (1996) compared the roles of nurses and alternate healers using the strategies of interviewing, participant observation, and analysis of books, music, and other artifacts related to healing. Magilvy et al. (1987) answered the question of "what it is like to be a teenager in a town in Colorado" by conducting interviews with parents, teachers, and teenagers, participant observation of teenagers, and analysis of secondary epidemiological data.

The use of triangulation involves more than just aggregating data (Silverman, 1993). The data from each source must be used to judge the validity of the data obtained from the other sources. Morse (1984), for example, found that by reviewing postnatal documentation and clinic records, she was able to understand the conflicts between the practices of breast-feeding advocated by the hospital and the actual practices that she observed and that were reported to her by the Fiji mothers.

Not all ethnographers stay within the above framework. Others add quantitative measures to the ethnographic strategies to triangulate even further. For example, Dreher and Hayes (1993) studied child development in Jamaica, using a participant observation approach and standardized measures of child development to study the long-term effect of use of cannabis perinatally. The ethnographic participant observations helped to refine the language of the quantitative instruments and increase their relevancy for the project. Likewise, the quantitative information provided support for the ethnographic findings from participant observation and interviews. This is an illustration of the use of multiple methods to study a single event—in this case, child development. The investigators moved back and forth between qualitative and quantitative methods in both data collection and data analysis.

Another example of using quantitative data to validate ethnographic data and vice versa is our own study (Roper & Shapira, 1999) on agitation in Alzheimer's patients. First, through ethnographic participant observation, we learned what questions were important in the lives of the nurses caring for Alzheimer's patients. As a result of these findings, we used open-ended interviewing of nurses as well as quantitative measures of depression, anxiety, and burden. We compared concepts that were identified in the interviews to the findings from the quantitative measures and our participant observation activities.

In sum, triangulation in ethnographic research usually occurs at the data collection and analysis level. The three strategies used in ethnography—participant observation, interviews, and examination of existing documents—provide a natural framework for triangulation.

THE RESONANCE OF NURSING PRACTICE WITH ETHNOGRAPHY

The practice of nursing is a complex, interactive process that occurs within diverse contexts. Research is needed that will provide direction for practice and insights into the context, the people, and the interactions of practice (Wilson, 1989). Ethnographic research methods can provide those insights. Parallels exist between ethnography and the nursing process.

For example, observation is an integral part of the nursing process within the context of health care delivery. In fact, the nursing process begins and ends with observation. Nurses use observational skills to gather data on the patient's condition, reflect on their observations to formulate the nursing assessment, and validate their assessment, whether with the patient, the family, or other staff or through the use of existing records, laboratory reports, physician's notes, or other documents, such as diagnostic tests and procedures. They develop a plan of care based upon the findings of the assessment. Nurses are both observers and participants in the health care environment as they interact with the patients and families to discover how individuals cope with illness and learn methods to enhance health. Nurses do all of this while maintaining a level of objectivity that ensures greater validity and reliability in their practice.

A similar pattern exists in ethnographic research. Field (1989) identified four similarities between investigators who conduct ethnographic research and nurses in clinical practice. First, nurses are good at interacting with people in a variety of circumstances. Ethnographers must also be able to interact with multiple participants in their studies in order to collect valid and reliable data. Second, nurses are careful listeners who are attentive to both verbal and nonverbal communication. Being a good listener is a must for ethnographers. Third, nurses observe and interpret on several levels at the same time—taking into account simultaneous factors present in the specific situation. In ethnography, the researcher does the same *and* is expected to document both the observation and the interpretation of the observation in a manner that is retrievable so that it can be further analyzed and conclusions can be drawn from it. Last, both nurses and researchers using ethnographic methods practice an intentional use of "self" called *reflexivity*. This involves being deliberately aware of oneself, one's responses, and one's internal state in relation to a specific situation and at the same time attempting to understand the patient and the situation. Psychiatric nurses in particular are skilled in reflexivity in their interactions with patients. Similarly, nurse ethnographers reflexively uncover nursing issues and meanings related to specific phenomena in patient care situations, talking to themselves as well as to others in order to construct the experience of the participants' worlds (Street, 1992). Reflexivity allows nurses to become aware of their role as ethnographers and to identify biases and their potential influence on the data and the interpretation of the data.

Ethnographic techniques reveal the meaningful way that nurses think and act within the framework of their lives. These are particularly useful in studies on how health and illness are perceived by both patients and nurses. The method uncovers taken-for-granted normal routines and the "contradictions between intent, meaning and action" (Street, 1992, p. 11). Street found that participant observation methods uncover the richness of nursing practice in this way. "To experience the awesome complexity of clinical nursing practice is to spend time in the swamp; to lay aside preconceived expectations and unexamined habits; to reject mythical thinking and easy solutions to well-known questions" (p. 15).

SUMMARY

In this chapter, we presented an overview of the ethnographic methods of participant observation, interviews, and review of available documents. The similarities between the methods of ethnography and nursing were identified. Criteria for the conduct of ethnographic participant observation were explained, and the levels or roles of participant observation activities were reviewed. The use of triangulation as a means of validating ethnographic research was described. Finally, the similarities between the methods of ethnography and nursing were identified. The important information to be remembered from this chapter by the researcher new to the ethnography is the following:

- Nurses are "naturals" at ethnography. The techniques that were learned in Nursing 101 parallel the ethnographic process, including participant observation, asking questions, and considering information about the patient obtained from other sources (existing documents). This does not mean that nurses can conduct ethnographic studies without additional information and training.

- In ethnography, the researcher is the instrument for data collection. The roles of participant-as-observer and observer-as-participant are those recommended for ethnographers, but you may move back and forth among the four roles during your study. It is not recommended that either the participant-only or the observer-only role be used by itself in the context of ethnographic research. Each level of participant observation has its own set of advantages and disadvantages. Most researchers move among the four levels during the conduct of a study. It is important as part of the reflexivity process (the use of self) to know which role is being assumed.

- Identifying the dimensions of time, place, social circumstances, language, intimacy, consensus, and bias is important to the successful conduct of ethnographic research.

- Interviewing can be formal or informal. Both types of interviews use open-ended questions.

- Existing data consist of documents that can be used to further understand your research question.

- Use triangulation when you need to strengthen the validity of your data and findings or when you are studying complex phenomena. Triangulation can be achieved by using the three data collection strategies—participant observation, interviewing, and examination of existing documents—and checking their findings against each other. Researchers can also triangulate by using more than one theoretical framework or analysis method, or including relevant quantitative measures.

3

HEADWORK AND FOOTWORK

What You Do Before Writing the Proposal

Where ask is have, where seek is find, where knock is open wide.
Christopher Smart, *A Song to David*
(1763, stanza 77; cited in Bartlett, 1968, p. 444a)

In this chapter, we review some general issues related to activities that need to be done before completing your research proposal. We discuss identifying the research question, assessing your level of knowledge about the subject, making contact with gatekeepers of organizations or groups where you wish to conduct your study, and assessing and obtaining the time and money needed to conduct the study.

IDENTIFY YOUR RESEARCH QUESTION

Identifying the research question is probably the most important aspect of preparing to conduct research (Brink & Wood, 1994). The research question will determine the methodology and guide the rest of your study. If it truly reflects what you want to do, all other aspects of your study will be consistent with the question. If, however, it does not accurately reflect what you intend to do in your project, then you will be in big trouble down the road. So take the time to ask yourself what you really want to learn from your study. Unlike traditional ethnography, in which the researcher entered the field with minimal direction, focused ethnography requires direction in terms of your research question.

In most focused ethnographies, and in qualitative, descriptive, and exploratory study designs in general, a first-level or "what" question is appropriate. First-level questions, though they may seem simplistic, are very complex and ultimately result in detailed information that cannot obtained from standard quantitative measures (Brink & Wood, 1994).

We find that nurses who are having difficulty writing a research proposal tend not to have their research question identified in a satisfactory manner. Often nurses prefer not to ask a first-level question because they perceive it as too easy. They much prefer asking a question whose answer is a yes or a no. One of the research questions for our agitation study (Roper & Shapira, 1999) was: "What are the characteristics of Alzheimer's disease (AD) patients whom nurses identify as agitated?" Very clearly, this was a first-level question requiring descriptive methods and analysis. The answer to that question was presented in terms of the demographic characteristics, as well as the behaviors, of AD patients whom nursing staff perceived as agitated.

A first-level clinical question that could be used for either inpatients or ambulatory care patients might be: "What are the methods used by psychiatric nurses to get psychiatric inpatients to take their psychotropic medication?" If we already knew what the methods were, a second-level question might be: "What is the relationship between the type of method used by psychiatric nurses and degree of success in getting psychiatric patients to take their medication?" Magilvy et al. (1987) asked the first-level question: "What is it like to be a teenager in a town in Colorado?"

Depending on the subject matter, a comparative or "what is the relationship between" question may be required (Brink & Wood, 1994). The study conducted by Dreher and Hayes (1993) focused on a second-level question in that it explored the relationship between a child's development and the mother's use of cannabis perinatally.

In our own agitation study (Roper & Shapira, 1999), a second-level question was: "What is the relationship between AD patient characteristics and the nurses' description of agitation?" The question was answered with comparative methods and correlation statistical analysis. We explored the relationship of patients' age, length of illness, and hospitalization to nurses' descriptions of agitation.

Third-level questions focus on *why* a phenomenon exists. Because you are using ethnographic methods, a third-level question is probably not appropriate.

Because your question is so important to the rest of your study, we strongly recommend the book by Brink and Wood (1994), which will further assist you with the process of defining your question. In addition, we offer a few suggestions:

- Ask the question you want to ask and not someone else's. This will save you much grief later on in the research process when you discover that the project you are designing is not the one you had in mind when you started working on your idea. You may lose interest in the study as a result.

- Talk with others about your project. Try to find a colleague who you trust to be honest with you and will give you both positive and negative feedback. Consult with researchers who have conducted studies in your area of interest. This process of interaction will help you define your question.

- Consult diverse sources for ideas: your experience, the research literature, and contemporary sources such as the arts and literature. In qualitative research, you want to have an open mind when you begin to explore your subject matter. Exploring a variety of sources may contribute to your openness.

- Give a lot of thought to the research question. Making sure it is right will save misery later on.

ASSESS YOUR LEVEL OF
KNOWLEDGE ABOUT THE SUBJECT

A second step is to determine what is known about your subject area. Though you want to conduct an ethnography with an open mind, you will be expected to be an expert on your subject or an expert in your methodology to obtain the information needed for your study. The question is, Do you study something you know a lot about or something you know little about? We cannot answer that question definitively. What you will read in the rest of this book may help you make the decision. For example, if you want to study in an area that you know something about, what kinds of issues have to be addressed, such as bias, that may influence validity and reliability in data collection and data analysis? Or is this a subject that requires an insider view, and are you studying it because your knowledge would be an asset to the research? Analyze what you objectively know about your research problem. If it is a problem related to your work experience, do others share it? Be open to opinions and attitudes other than your own.

If it is a topic or area that is completely new to you, what do you need to do to write a proposal on the subject? Perhaps pilot study data will fill the gap. Certainly talking to others about your idea and talking to those who know the subject or work in that specific field will be of assistance. After completion of our study on agitation in AD (Roper & Shapira, 1999), JS was interested in studying agitation in an acute care setting. To determine if agitation was an issue for critical care nurses, she had to consult with the staff in the intensive care units. She let them tell her about the problems in acute care. As a result, she learned that agitation in patients following surgery was a major problem.

It may also help to do some introspection about the subject. Your motives may potentially bias your study. It is not unusual for nurses, interested in research but neophytes to the process, to consult us with "There is this wonderful tool I want to use in my research." They have no idea how to use the tool or what to use it for, but they have attached themselves to it as if it were their best friend.

Or perhaps you want to "prove" something. You have an idea that if the nurses would just change a procedure, then care would be improved. With qualitative research and quantitative as well, you don't "prove" anything. You support your ideas and hypotheses, or you find no support for them. So if "proving" something is your motivation, consider refocusing your question and purpose. Explore your motivations related to conducting the study, and try to objectify your intentions through a good research question that can be answered.

You need to learn what others have said about your topic. Review of the literature indicates what has been done on the topic and what is missing. One reason to conduct qualitative research and focused ethnography on a subject is that there is little or no formal information on it. For example, in the literature on restraints and seclusion, there has traditionally been little information about *how* a patient ends up in restraints and/or locked seclusion. Almost all the literature when Roper (Roper & Anderson, 1991) conducted her study on the process of restraints/ seclusion was related to figures on who went into restraints, how long they stayed, their diagnosis, their age, and the reason for their hospitalization. Thus, she designed a qualitative study to answer the research question: "What is the process by which patients are placed in restraints and/or locked seclusion room on an intensive care psychiatric inpatient ward?"

Likewise, when we were preparing to do our study of agitation, we found that the concept of agitation was poorly defined in the literature. There was agreement that AD patients were often agitated and that agitation presented management problems to caregivers, but there was no information on the perception of the caregiver in relation to agitation or on how the agitation affected the caregiver and ultimately influenced management. These are complex issues in the day-to-day management of the care of the AD patient. Often, then, the lack of knowledge in the research literature about a subject matter is the impetus for the research question.

Clinicians can provide you with much information about your subject and help to clarify the research subject and question. For example, when JS talked with critical care clinicians, she found that nurses and physicians were confounded by the problem of agitation and behavioral problems in intensive care units. Medications often did not help and in fact sometimes compounded the problem. The more she learned about this problem, the more it became apparent that agitation in critical care areas was very important to nurses. Even though studies had been conducted on behavior problems in intensive care units, a missing piece of information was the interpretation and action of the nurses in the delivery of care. Ethnographic research was one way to understand the phenomenon.

Consider the possibility of collaborating with a nurse colleague or someone from the professional team in health care. The advantage of sharing the study with other health care professionals is a distribution of the workload. The headwork and footwork can be divided between the team members. Also, enlisting the help of someone from the agency where you are going to conduct the study can be a major advantage. Their participation may facilitate the access to the population that you need to conduct the study. A disadvantage to team research is that you have to take extra steps to ensure that all members of the team are conducting the study in the same way and that the roles of team members are clearly understood by all.

CONTACTING THE GATEKEEPERS

Before you write the proposal, you need to meet with the gatekeepers, the people who allow you access to the setting and to the population, in the settings that are appropriate for the conduct the study, about their willingness to allow you in their setting. If you are a member of that setting, you may or may not have problems, or your problems may be very different.

If you want access to a setting where you are unknown, you must now do both head and footwork. You must find the gatekeepers in order to begin the negotiations on allowing their staff and patients to be participants in your study. Do this step early in your study development. You should be able to talk to the gatekeepers about your study in some detail. They need to know the time needed to conduct the study, what staff and patients are involved in the project, and whether the study represents risks, hazards, or an inconvenience for patients. If this is a medical center, you start with the director of nurses or the person in charge of nursing research. That person can then identify others who may be helpful in negotiating the system. Heed the advice of these staff members. Their job is to protect the agency and persons under their jurisdiction from undue stress and disorder. They are generally very protective of their patients and staff. They are suspicious of outsiders, so you may have to contact more than one setting before you find an agency that welcomes your study.

If you are conducting a study in the community, the same principles apply, but the routes to and through the gatekeeper differ. For example, Cook and de Mange (1995) did both headwork and footwork for 1 year to gain access to a Native American group. They provide the reader with a detailed account of their experiences.

There are different levels of gatekeepers. In the formal organization, one level is the staff members who approve research proposals. Another level is the nursing supervisor, nursing manager, clinic director, or service chief who is responsible for persons under his or her supervision. You may have to make several calls or get referrals from colleagues about potential facilities and names of staff to contact. For example, as the person at my facility responsible for nursing research, JR is frequently contacted by staff outside and inside the setting about who is the best person to talk to about a project that is being formalized as a proposal. So talk to the gatekeepers—be honest and open with them about what you think you want to do (remember, you probably do not have a written proposal at this point). A good example of the chain of gatekeepers you may have to go through was provided by Mayo (1992). To access a sample of black working women, the ethnographer had to contact community agencies, personnel directors, occupational health nurses, and her professional colleagues.

If you are an insider to the organization or field site, you may have other issues to deal with if you want to study something in your own organization. Just what issues will depend on your position in the organization and exactly what you want to do in your research. Institutions would probably not be comfortable with a staff member studying other staff members whom they work with every day. In fact, some years ago, a research and development office rejected a project because investigators were studying their own staff. Even though this was a quantitative study and a system was developed for anonymity and confidentiality of responses, the office still believed that staff studying staff created a bias that no one could overlook, even on a paper-and pencil questionnaire. If you are an authority figure in the organization and you want to study a situation in the organization involving staff that you supervise, you may also hit an insurmountable barrier. You need to discuss these issues with the gatekeepers. Carr (1996) reported that he had no problems accessing the members and staff of the "HIV Hotel" because he was a member of the health delivery team at a major AIDS clinic.

In Chapter 5, we discuss in detail more strategies for gaining access. Suffice it to say at this point that even early in your project development it may be wise to also contact the formal gatekeepers for the organization, society, and culture—those persons who have the authority to allow you entrance to a facility, tribe, clinic, school, or other group or organization. In complex organizations where there are layers of "authority" people, you may need to start querying who gives access early in the study process. If staff are involved in your study, they can still say no, even if the authorities have given you approval. Again, work through the system so that this does not happen. You do not want to write a proposal and then not be able to conduct the study because you cannot gain access to a group or organization.

The research department in complex organizations may be able to help you decide whom to talk to about access. In fact, you may have to get a signature of approval as part of the research review process. If there is a nurse-researcher or a nurse in charge of research in the organization, then contact that person for the appropriate information. Nurses who do research tend to keep in touch with one another, so if you do not know anyone in the specific organization and are stuck getting information, then try a researcher that you do know. Ask that person for a contact person in the organization where you want to conduct your study. Keeping lines of communication open with the organization is key to the process. Organizations and cultures are protective of their subjects—they have mechanisms in place to protect the staff, patients, and families from outsiders who are not known. The gatekeepers do not know if you can be trusted to work with the members of their organization. They do not know if you will exploit them for your own benefit or even lie about them in your reports. Set up contacts that will facilitate entry into the organization or group. Some organizations even have rules about nonstaff conducting research in their setting. If you run into this problem, you will have to finesse your way into the setting. You may have to develop the study in association with someone on staff or obtain a without-salary position to qualify to conduct the study. You must check the rules with the research department.

TIME AND MONEY

Will you have the time to conduct this study? If you are a student, you need to project your time allotment, as you will want to obtain your degree within a reasonable period of time. What about your other classes, if any? Your family obligations? Vacations? How many hours in the day do you have to devote to the study? Is the study site close, or do you drive an hour or more to get to the study site? Or do you have multiple study sites? All of these issues must be taken into consideration when planning your study.

As a working, employed person outside your home, you have to ask yourself similar questions. Will your current job release you to conduct research? If they will release you, for how much time? How much time can you devote to the project after your work hours? Is that feasible? Are your subjects available during your work hours only? What are your family obligations? Are they negotiable?

Always allow yourself more time to do the study than you actually project. When studies start, there are always unforeseeable delays, such as earthquakes or even less drastic events, that are totally out of your control. Be reasonable with your time projections, but always expect the unexpected, and try to build in a little extra time to complete your study. This is always important but particularly of concern if you do not have much money to support the conduct of your study.

Part of your headwork is developing a budget for both your time and other resources needed—particularly money. Not only do you not want to run out of time, but you want to have enough other resources to conduct the research in a reasonable and timely fashion. So as you think about your time, you must also think about money and additional help you will need. If you do decide that you need support in terms of funding, you will want to develop a budget for the allocation of the money so that you use the funds within the time specified and according to the time projections related to fund distribution. Developing a budget is usually part of the research proposal package for funding. The package contains the guidelines and requirements for that particular funding source. What is not in the guidelines is any indication of how to develop the budget with real money. Again, you will have to consult either the staff at the agency where you are processing your application or other researchers who have written budgets and will offer you their expertise. One thing you must do with a budget is break it down into units (usually years) and activities. For example, if you have funds for a research assistant and you have indicated to the funding source that you will hire the research assistant within the first quarter of your study, then you will need to do that. If you do not hire the research assistant until the third or fourth quarter, you may lose the first- and second-quarter funds!

Last, but certainly not least, is the issue of funding. Can you do the study without outside funding? This is a two-edged sword in many ways. For pilot studies, you may be able to find support from local agencies such as health associations or professional organizations. Pilot studies may be less attractive to the major funding sources. You may have a project that must be funded before you can conduct it. However, you may also decide that even though the project should be done with funding, you will not go for the money because you do not want to be hassled with the process and you can finesse conducting the study while working at your current job. You do not want to be bothered with the time and effort it takes to write the research grant and the waiting period. You just want to do your study. That is okay, but later in your career, you may find that you need a track record of funding for that new position or for promotion. So search your motivation, once again, and be true to yourself and to your future before you say, "I can do this study without funding."

SUMMARY

In this chapter, we have discussed the activities that need to be done either before writing the proposal or as soon as you have a draft of a study in hand. Part of what is required is thinking and planning, and part is making contacts needed for the actual conduct of your study. The key points to remember from this chapter are the following:

- The headwork associated with conducting research and participant observation involves determining your research question, assessing your knowledge of the subject, and querying yourself regarding time and other resources needed to do the study.

- Footwork involves contacting gatekeepers of the area(s) where you want to do your study.

- Consider the issues of time and your funding needs before you start a project.

4

WRITING THE RESEARCH PROPOSAL

Good words are worth much, and cost little.
George Herbert, *Jacula Prudentum* (1651;
cited in Bartlett, 1968, p. 324a)

Early anthropological accounts of ethnographies were not directed by a research proposal, at least not the formalized written proposal required by most agencies today. If you are conducting a study in the Western world and using institutions, agencies, and health care settings of various types, a written proposal is now mandated before agency approval for conducting a study can be obtained. It was possible, once, to go into the field with your curiosity and some questions to guide your field experience. Now, for most studies that are conducted by nurses within the Western world, formal written proposals are a must. Certainly, if funding is attached to a study, whoever holds the purse strings must be provided with a written document that outlines your research.

In this chapter, we describe the formalization of your research through the written proposal. Most agencies have institutional review boards (IRBs) that have established criteria, forms, and processes for proposal submission, review, and approval. You must check with the

39

agency about the requirements. This is part of the process of obtaining permission to conduct a study. The IRB is one form of gatekeeping for the agency. Also in this chapter we will review the requirements for proposals that are written for funding purposes.

Several books and articles describe the headings and required content of the research proposal (Brink & Wood, 1994; Burgess, 1984b; Cohen, Knafl, & Dzurec, 1993; Fetterman, 1989; Leininger, 1985; Morse & Field, 1995; Sandelowski, Davis, & Harris, 1989). If you are reading this book, we hope that you have had an introductory course on research so that you have some familiarity with the content of a proposal. We strongly recommend the Brink and Wood (1994) text as a source for beginning researchers. It is extremely reader friendly and full of practical information related to designing your proposal.

Despite the resources that are usually available to the neophyte researcher, this chapter is included to give you an overview of the "usual" content, as well as those specific needs of qualitative research in a proposal. The "usual" content is presented with the caveat that you must check with your organization to make sure you are using the proper format, including headings, on the proposal.

PROPOSAL CONTENT

In a formal proposal, there is usually a narrative section written as part of the proposal packet, as well as title pages, abstract, budget, timetable, resources, and consent forms that are appended to the narrative. Instructions and even examples may be provided to assist you in completing the required information. Be sure to follow whatever instructions are supplied. JR has seen proposals returned to the investigator because the headings were incorrect on the consent form or page numbers were exceeded or copies were submitted when the original was requested. Agencies are very particular about their guidelines and do not publish them to have them ignored. Sometimes you may need the assistance of a "translator" to understand them, so if you do not understand the instructions, ask for help from someone within the agency.

The narrative section headings vary by institution but generally include the information listed in Table 4.1 and discussed below. Remember that these headings were initially established for quantitative re-

---

TABLE 4.1   Research Proposal Headings

---

1. Aims of your study (short and long term)
   Research questions
   Hypotheses

2. A background section that includes
   Rationale
   Literature review
   Preliminary studies
   Your background

3. Significance

4. Methodology
   Design
   Subjects
   Tools and instruments
   Protection of human subjects
   Data analysis

---

search. You may have some problems fitting the content appropriate for qualitative research into a quantitative framework. There are no standards, however, for qualitative research in terms of headings for proposal submission.

The content related to the headings in Table 4.1, once on your word-processing program, can be shifted around to meet the specific requirements of different review boards. It is not unusual to have to change formats for different review agencies. We once revised the same proposal five times for different funding sources. The content was not different, but the way the content was organized changed. Each of the above major headings in Table 4.1 is briefly discussed. General information about what is required in each section is explained, and then the information related specifically to ethnographic research is identified.

AIMS OF YOUR STUDY

In this section, describe what you want to do with your study, and enumerate specific objectives; identify hypotheses if appropriate. This section sets the frame for the rest of your proposal. Your research question is not always stated explicitly, but it can be. Because the research question directs the rest of the research, the specificity of this section will reflect whether you have really identified your research problem. If the aim is vague and wordy, you probably have not clearly focused on your research question. The reader will know immediately if this is so. Remember that this section is the one reviewers will see first, so make it clear and concise. Most reviewers read several proposals and do not like reading jargon or needless verbiage.

To hypothesize or not to hypothesize in ethnographic research—that is the question! Ethnographic research is a type of qualitative research and as such is a method that produces findings not arrived at by usual quantification and statistical procedures (Strauss & Corbin, 1990). In general, ethnography offers "thick" descriptions of the understanding and practices of a group of people. Also, ethnographic research, due to the richness of the information, may raise questions that lead to hypothesized relationships or point out directions for further research. Because the goal of ethnographic research is to discover salient features through the gathering of information, hypotheses are generally not postulated when the study is designed. Rather, ethnography is an inductive process in which the course of events, rather than the researcher's preconceived ideas, dictates the research (Golander, 1992). The concern of some qualitative researchers is that designing a qualitative study around a core hypothesis will prevent the learning process from occurring. Yet ethnographic researchers do know quite a bit before they go into the field. They have read materials by others who have studied or worked with a similar group of people. For example, you might study health care practices of community members with access to a variety of health care settings and wish to learn (among other things) who uses these facilities. On the basis of previous reading, you predict that distance from home will influence the decision of where to obtain care. You then formulate the hypothesis that "people use the health care facility that is closest to their home."

In this day of funding requirements, hypotheses are often expected in every proposal. In academia, professors may require you to articulate your hunches about your subject area in terms of hypotheses. These hunches or hypotheses remain fluid in ethnographic studies to allow for changes in your thinking after encountering the specific realities of actual fieldwork. If you cannot write hypotheses, then the research question(s) will serve to guide your research. Follow the requirements of your facility, the institution where you are conducting the research, and the funding agency guidelines regarding hypotheses. We recommend consulting Brink and Wood (1994) for more explicit advice on your research question and hypothesis formulation.

In total, this section of your proposal is the marketing pitch for your study; it should hook the reader into your study. It is important that it be detailed but not wordy, clear but not redundant. For example, you want to convince the reader that the issues identified in the aim or aims are important to nursing and health care.

For your specific ethnographic study, begin with the initial question that prompted your study. Then move on to orienting definitions specific to your study. Include both short- and long-term aims, as well as a brief overview of the background of the study (Sandelowski et al., 1989). An example of a short-term aim is to spend 1 month at the study site as an observer more than a participant in order to collect some specific data and also to learn about where you need to be to observe the phenomenon being studied.

Burgess (1984b) and Cohen et al. (1993) suggested the inclusion of a theoretical/conceptual framework for your research question. The framework assists you in determining the kinds of questions you need to address, as well as the kinds of data that are needed to answer the question.

BACKGROUND

This section includes current and classic literature on your subject. Reviewers look for the most current works related to the topic and expect that you know them by citing them. Weave the information from the literature into the schema of your study. What is the relevance of the cited studies for your study? Do they support your project, or do you have to defend your research idea by pointing out the differences and build from there? If there are classic, not necessarily current writings on your subject, be sure to cite them and place them within the perspective of your study. For instance, in this book, we cite both new and old references—both have a place within this portion of the proposal, in order to show the reader how much you know about your subject matter. Many citations will be research-related papers and books on your topic. Sometimes, however, you may need to include purely theoretical or clinical/experiential papers to support what you want to do. For example, in our agitation study (Roper & Schapira, 1999), we included references that detailed nursing interventions for patients who were agitated. These were not research papers, yet they contributed to our proposal by demonstrating that management strategies for agitated patients were available. What was missing was empirical study of the nursing caregiver perspective on agitation and use of the methods.

Present information that explains why and how this study came into being. Was it a clinical question or a question prompted by literature? Just what is the background of the study?

Included in this section is *your* background, as well as the literature that forms the background on the topic. A description about you is required: your previous experience related to the topic and your publications, if any, that strengthen your ability to conduct this study. If you have only clinical experience, describe that. You may have to identify a mentor who will assist you with the actual conduct of the study if research is new to you. It has been speculated by Morse (1991) that funding agencies are really funding the ethnographic (or qualitative) investigator rather than the project. Inexperienced researchers must have the active support of consultants and advisors to increase their chances of being funded. Your strengths related to the topic and the methodology are presented in this background section. In sum, in this section, you answer the question: Which of your experiences qualify you to conduct the study?

Preliminary study data also go in this section. It is important, especially if this is a funding agency for which you are writing the proposal, to have pilot or preliminary data that you can share. The reviewer will know that there is some substance to what you propose to do if you can back it up with supporting data.

Important to reviewers is the fact that you have substantiated in the background the need for the ethnographic methodology and your expertise to conduct this type of qualitative study.

SIGNIFICANCE

In the significance section, you must make a case for the importance of your study—usually by describing possible uses of the findings. You must let the reader know that this study is more than just a fishing expedition. Funding agencies have targeted topics that are important to them. It is in your interest to relate your study to those topics if possible. Funding agencies may also want to know how you plan to disseminate your findings. If the study is important, then you need to know how you can share this information with those who might use the findings to their benefit.

You can begin by reiterating statistics regarding the magnitude of the problem you are studying and then describe the potential effect of your findings on the problem. If statistics are not available or appropriate for your particular problem/study, then you must discuss relevancy to, for example, patient care issues or health care delivery enhancement. Tie your study to the important issues associated with the problem that your project addresses.

For ethnographic research, this section addresses the need to obtain the information proposed in the study by this qualitative method. Assure the reviewer that no other methodology is appropriate. Remember that conducting an ethnography is expensive because of the time involved in both data collection and analysis. Many agencies want results yesterday and may be reluctant to support research that will take months to years to complete. Also, agencies, because of their familiarity with quantitative and not qualitative research, may be uncomfortable with the methodology and may have concerns about whether it is scientific. Your job is to convince them, in the significance section, that the effort will result in information that is important to health care.

METHODOLOGY

The methodology section of a proposal either makes or breaks approval and/or funding. You may think that the methodology is clear, but rethink that position before you finalize your proposal. It may be clear to you because you have been ruminating, rewriting, and "playing" with methodology for some time as you have developed your proposal. But the reader has not been there with you while you have gone through this process. Therefore, you must make this section extremely clear and detailed. Do not assume that your reader can follow the steps in your methodology. You must state those steps!

Your methodology must reflect back on your aims, research questions, or hypotheses. The methodology must be appropriate to the purpose. You do not want to describe a methodology that clearly will not answer your research question.

For your ethnographic research, being clear about your methods is even more important. You may have to include a step-by-step outline of participant observation. More definitions and explanations are necessary because, remember, the reviewer probably knows little or nothing about ethnography. You must clarify and justify your plan. Even though you have probably defended the methodology earlier in your study, state the justification again. Chart for the reviewer the initial direction of the proposal, but also inform him or her that there is flexibility in the plan. Explain that ethnography is driven by what happens in the field and not by preconceived ideas.

The *design* of your study tells the reader in a few words what to expect in the rest of the methodology section. If you are conducting a study that compares variables, then you have an experimental design of some sort. If you are describing phenomena, then you may be using a descriptive, exploratory design. The design sets the framework for the rest of the methodology description.

The design of ethnographic research is usually exploratory or descriptive. If you include other data collection methods, such as standardized tools, then the study may be both descriptive and comparative. Again, the research question drives the rest of the study, so if you have identified in the research question issues that cannot be investigated using participant observation techniques alone, you need to address how you will collect information related to those issues.

You must describe your *subjects or participants* in this section: who they will be, where they will come from, how many there will be, how you will obtain access to them, and inclusion/exclusion criteria. In ethnographic research, the number of subjects is not nearly as important as availability and willingness of subjects to be observed or interviewed

Situations may be more important than subjects. In that case, you need to identify those situations and how feasible it is for you to be a participant/observer in the situations. As a woman, you may not be able to obtain access to totally male situations; men may be restricted from strictly female interactions.

Sampling in ethnographic research is usually theoretical or purposive, so even if you cannot come up with numbers for the proposal, you can define who the subjects might be, where you expect to locate them, and criteria for selection in your sample.

Tools and instruments are described in detail. If you are using both ethnographic and quantitative measures, you need to describe each strategy in detail.

Because you are the instrument in ethnographic research, the reader needs to know your exact role. Are you participant, observer, or both? Describe your relationship to the situation that you are observing. Acknowledge reliability and validity issues, and state how you are going to address them. Address the issue of bias in particular. See Chapters 6 and 8 for detailed information.

If you have included a quantitative component to enhance the validation of your ethnographic data through triangulation, then you need, in addition to describing the tools/instruments, the psychometrics of the measures. Describe the purpose of the tools, when the tools will be administered, and how they are related to aims and questions or hypotheses of the study. A table is a concise way of organizing this information for the reader. It can include, for example, your variable to be measured, the instrument that measures it, and data collection points for the measure.

Protection of human subjects may be addressed in this section. In qualitative research, you may or may not have an informed-consent form process, but you will still need to describe how your subjects will be protected. Agencies have their own standard forms to complete for human consent. Always included in such guidelines are the description of study, procedures used in the study, risks and benefits of the study for the patient, and telephone number of the researcher.

DATA ANALYSIS

Identify, in this section, the *specific strategies* you intend to use to analyze the data from the study. In ethnographic research proposals, you will describe how you will manage the data while you are in the field collecting data and after you have completed your field experience. Share with the reader what specific steps you will take to reduce your data to a reasonable size. You may not be able to detail all the steps because, after all, you may not have others' research findings, which would necessarily help you design the analysis. But a few basic ideas that you can describe to the reader of this proposal will increase the perception of you as a competent qualitative researcher. Reviewers of qualitative research look for the investigators' competency in the methodology, as well as the presentation of the ideas, assumptions, sampling, data collection, and analysis (Cohen et al., 1993). If you lack competency in the specific methodology, perhaps you can conduct a pilot study using the qualitative strategy or employ the assistance of a consultant or mentor who has the expertise.

OTHER ASPECTS OF THE PROPOSAL

When you write the proposal, use simple, clear language and avoid verbosity. Make your proposal easy for the reader to follow, and describe it so completely that the reviewers can visualize the process. Detail clearly for the reviewers how validity and reliability will be established.

If you are including quantitative data sources, you will need to know what to do with those data. A statistician consulted early in your proposal development can assist you in determining the correct form of analysis. A paragraph or so must be devoted to power analysis in any quantitative study component to determine sample size.

Descriptions are written for each of the hypotheses (again, if any) that is subjected to analysis.

A timetable that outlines your data collection is helpful in your proposal. Some funding agencies require such a document. If you are conducting the study as a team, you also need to specify the roles of the team members. Tell the reviewer what you are going to do, why you are going to do it, and how you will analyze and report the study within some organizational or conceptual framework. It is important to build a case for what you want to do and then explain why the specific method is appropriate to that aim.

Budgeting is often identified as a problem in funding proposals. If you do require a budget (and most studies should), it should be detailed and all items justified as to their need. Make sure you read the guidelines of the funding agency to determine if they have limits on total amounts and restrictions on what can be on a budget. Consult with people who do budgets or with other researchers who have completed budgets (and been funded) before you complete your own.

To be submitted as part of the proposal packet are letters of support from the agencies where you will conduct your research. These are important documents that are carefully reviewed by the readers of the study. Readers want to be assured that the study can be conducted at the indicated site and that a cooperative and supportive spirit is demonstrated by the agency.

In sum, your proposal, in whatever format, must be an integrated whole. You must begin and end with the same aims and hypotheses. What you have said in the background section must be related to the beginning and end. The methodology has to be appropriate for the task and described in detail so that the reader will not have to guess about any aspect of tools, data collection, or subjects.

ISSUES RELATED TO THE
ETHNOGRAPHIC PROPOSAL

According to Burgess (1984b), most nonqualitative proposals traditionally look very linear. In reality, especially in ethnographic research, the actual conduct of the study is nonlinear, with the interaction between the researcher and researched influencing the course of the research. JR initiated the conduct of her doctoral research using exchange as the theoretical framework, but it became evident early in the observation portion of the study that exchange was not appropriate for the psychiatric inpatient setting. JR then had to seek a more appropriate conceptual basis for the study. Some flexibility is required when writing the ethnographic proposal. The aim is to tell the reader, particularly a funding agency, what is needed to get the funding, with enough flexibility built in so that modifications can be made as the need arises. Qualitative research methods are used when little is known about a phenomenon, so your proposal requirements may not be as exacting as those for quantitative studies (Sandelowski et al., 1989).

Ethnographic researchers are often concerned that their methodology may not be understood by reviewers or may be perceived as being not as rigorous as quantitative methods and that on account of this their studies or funding for their studies may not be approved. But Cohen et al. (1993) found that reviewers of qualitative grant proposals were able to recognize the salient issues related to these proposals and were able to give feedback to the researchers that was helpful. Reviewers look for much the same information here as in nonqualitative research: the scientific contribution of the study, the framework that guides the research, and the expertise of the proposal writers. A well-written ethnographic proposal that has significance for nursing is not overlooked by reviewers.

An emphasis on triangulation and the addition of a quantitative component to the proposal design and methodology potentially enhance the research and strengthen the outcomes. So whether you are looking to developing a purely ethnographic research study or are adding a quantitative portion to your qualitative study, the outlook for positive reviews has improved.

COMMON METHODOLOGICAL PROBLEMS

We now discuss some of the common methodological problems found in ethnographic research proposals. This information comes primarily from reviews of reports by funding agencies. Whether you are submitting your study for funding consideration or trying to satisfy the institutional IRB requirements, heed the comments that follow. These comments come from Bootzin, Sechrest, Scott, and Hannah (1992) and Cohen et al. (1993), as well as from our own experiences in writing proposals, teaching students the proposal-writing process, and being on groups that review research proposals.

In the *background* section of the proposal, make sure that you have important and relevant areas covered thoroughly. Although researchers with little or no knowledge of your subject area may review your proposal, you can be sure that someone on the review panel will be an expert on your topic and/or your methodology. You will not be able to slight this section of the proposal with jargon and quick overviews. This section should reflect your state of the knowledge on your subject, including opposing arguments.

Specific to the *methodology* are concerns about the design of the study. A most frequently identified problem has to do with variables that would confound the control and experimental groups. In ethnographic research, you may not face this dilemma; however, if you triangulate using quantitative methods, then you may have to address the confounding variables that *might* influence outcomes and what you are going to do about them. Loss of subjects due to attrition is also a problem in many studies, particularly quantitative. Again, you may have to address this qualitatively as well. What if the situation that you are studying changes or is modified in some way that influences your original research question? Though you may not be able to consider all possible contingencies, you must explain the more obvious. For example, suppose that you plan to study smoking in psychiatric inpatients but the policy at the agency where you are conducting your study changes and you suddenly find that all patients are now required to go outside to smoke. An artifact has been created, and you can no longer study this phenomenon in a naturalistic way. What happens to your research? Can you still study smoking in psychiatric patients if smoking is restricted? Do you look for another agency where smoking is not restricted, or do you change your research focus?

Lack of operational definitions regarding treatment or intervention conditions in experimental research is another methodological issue. In relation to ethnographic research, definitions may also be lacking that describe the way in which you are using specific strategies. For example, we have discussed in earlier chapters the lack of clarity regarding what ethnographic research is. Ethnography seems to be a concept that has some agreed-upon but varying meanings among social scientists. Perhaps that was appropriate in the earlier days of anthropology, but now the meaning of the term in the individual study must be explained. In this book, for example, we take the position that the use of participant observation, interviewing, and use of existing documentation is intrinsic to ethnographic research, whether by themselves or in combination with other methods.

Statistical analysis in the methodological section is another area that has been problematic for reviewers. When using statistics in your research, unless you are a statistical wizard, employ the assistance of a statistician early in your project. Where you are converting qualitative data to numbers, the assistance of a person familiar with this process may be helpful for making full use of your data.

Making sure that your sample is representative is a methodological issue that must be resolved in both qualitative and quantitative studies. In quantitative studies, it can be addressed by randomization strategies. In ethnographic studies, the researcher must justify the participant observation strategies. To observe the phenomena that you want, you must explain why and how your specific plan for participant observation strategies will achieve that goal.

Reliability and validity as methodological concerns are discussed in the chapter on data collection. Acknowledge in your proposal the reliability and validity issues and what you have done to ensure consistency and accuracy in data collection and data analysis. Depending upon whether you are reading discussions of ethnography or studies from naturalistic researchers, you will find a difference in their attitudes toward reliability and validity. You should describe the weaknesses of your study and how these will affect the outcomes. These strategies are discussed in some detail in the previous chapters. If you are using quantitative tools as well, you must address the respondent burden issues. Tools that take subjects a long time to complete may not be acceptable to review boards.

Concerns about *data collection* methods arise in both quantitative and qualitative studies. This section of your proposal must be explained very clearly for either type of study. Do not leave out any steps in data collection. The reader must be able to understand the process. Often ethnographic methodologies seem mysterious because they are hard to explain to the reader. You must, however, demystify the techniques and explain each step. In ethnographic research, you must also leave some room for flexibility in data collection because you are engaged in a learning process. So be as clear and concise as you can without jeopardizing the actual conduct of your study.

The *significance* section is important to all research. It should include how the findings will benefit the institution where the study will be conducted and perhaps the population of patients being studied as well. For example, many funding agencies have identified target populations for which they are most interested in funding research. So the significance should specifically address how the study will benefit that specific group. Another issue you might address in the significance section is the benefit for nursing.

SUMMARY

Writing the research proposal is a tedious but extremely important task. A written proposal of some sort will be required by most agencies. Remember to do the following when you write your research proposal:

- Ask the agency/setting where you propose to conduct your study about what kind of written proposal is required, and then follow their guidelines religiously.

- If you are interested in funding for your study, potential funding sources' guidelines must also be followed. If possible, attend conferences/workshops on grantsmanship, or consult with others who have submitted proposals for funding and were successful. Written materials on grantsmanship are also available.

- As qualitative research, focused ethnography requires some special attention in the proposal. Defining and clarifying your steps in the study, discussing your rationale for conducting the study and for using participant observation, and showing your awareness of the weaknesses and the reliability/validity issues related to your study will strengthen the proposal and increase the likelihood of approval.

5

GETTING YOUR FOOT
IN THE DOOR

Make haste; the better foot before.

Shakespeare, *King John (Act 4, Scene 2;*
cited in Bartlett, 1968, p. 237a)

The information in this chapter is based upon the assumption that you have completed the headwork and footwork discussed in Chapter 3 and are now ready to gain formal access to (a) the institution or setting where you want to conduct your participant observation research and (b) the group members and situations you want to observe for the understanding of behaviors, thoughts, and meanings ascribed to events in the setting. In most writing on ethnography, gaining access is presented as a complex process fraught with problems that are totally unexpected. A most dreaded event would be the disappearance of your problem or research question from the setting before you even get a chance to conduct the research. For instance, suppose you want to study smoking habits of psychiatric patients on an inpatient ward, but before you get to conduct the study, the institution adopts a "no smoking" policy and bans all smoking on inpatient wards. Or the phenomenon that is the subject of your research ceases to exist once you get into the setting.

The latter happened to JR when she was studying restraints and seclusion on an acute psychiatric ward. For a whole month after she entered the setting, patients were not placed in restraints or seclusion. Before that, restraints and seclusion had been used on a fairly regular basis. But fortunately, after the initial month, the use of restraints and seclusion did recur. If you find yourself in such a situation, continue your participant research, and perhaps try to find out the meaning to your participants of the *absence* of the events you intended to study. Or perhaps, as in the case of the smoking study, you can refocus the study.

Remember that gaining access to a facility and to your research participants is a process—something that does not just happen but must be worked through the specific organization or population. Every agency or organization has its own review and approval process for the conduct of research. You must determine early in your proposal development which system to review and approve proposed studies is used by the organization where you will conduct your study. Larger institutions have formalized processes that are driven by federal rules to protect human subjects. Smaller hospitals and clinics and less formal community-type settings may have more informal processes in place. For example, in some institutions you may have to present your study to a panel of clinical and administrative staff for approval to conduct your research rather than to a formal institutional review board (IRB). Or you may have to go through a number of steps to gain access to a group of people (Cook & de Mange, 1995).

This chapter describes IRB processes related to informed consent for human subjects and scientific merit reviews. It also discusses issues specific to getting approval for qualitative research and ethnographic studies. The last section of the chapter deals with the final step of getting your foot in the door: gaining access to the population and/or specific situation required for your study.

INSTITUTIONAL REVIEW BOARD PROCESSES

Reviews are conducted by IRBs to ensure the protection of human subjects and to determine the scientific merit of the proposed study. In these processes, a person or persons unconnected with your proposal review your study for human subjects protection and scientific merit. There are generally timetables to be adhered to in the IRB structure, so be sure to determine the specific method by which you submit your study for review and the time parameters. It facilitates the review process if the project is discussed with the nurse on the IRB committee or the person in charge of the review process—the chair of the department or chair of the research committee. These "contact persons" or "sponsors," as they are termed by Street (1992), will vary depending upon the situation. Street (1992) first contacted a nursing supervisor in the facility to which he wished to gain access, Germain (1979) contacted the director of nursing, and Preston (1997) contacted his institution's ethics committee. All these investigators then were referred to other key staff in order to gain access to the facility and staff. Hyland and Morse (1995) had to obtain permission from their university's IRB, a large mortuary firm, and two funeral parlor directors in one city in order to gain access to situations where they could learn about funeral directors. Perhaps one of the more lengthy processes is described by Cook and de Mange (1995). One year before entering a Native American community, the authors had to contact the Bureau of Indians Affairs for a list of Native American reservations, request permission from the specific tribal government for access to a specific reservation, and then get final local permission from the health care providers and the addiction program director at the reservation. In addition, the Indian Health Service required specific study information before access was allowed.

Some organizations that are affiliated with academia contract with their university's human subjects subcommittee to review the proposal for human subjects' protection. Then the institution reviews the proposal for scientific merit and approves or disapproves the protocol after receiving input from the university subcommittee. Committees may allow you to present your study verbally but not to be present for the final voting. Committees generally meet monthly, so you need to follow their guidelines for submission dates. Allow yourself plenty of time to get through the review process. Approval can be held up pending feedback from you for clarification. The review process can involve many unanticipated delays, so allow extra time for the unexpected. Committees are usually composed of staff from the organization who are investigators—a broad mix of clinicians and scientists. Larger organizations have a greater number of resources and are able to provide a cross section of disciplines on these committees. Increasingly, nurses have become a part of these review boards.

There may be a nursing research committee in larger, complex institutions. This group may be advisory to the larger IRB, or it may do its own review before submission to the IRB. It is just another process that is part of some institutions. You need to find out just what processes for review are required by the institution where you want to gain access.

PROTECTION OF HUMAN SUBJECTS

Even though there are basic rules on protection of human subjects, each IRB has its own forms and required information to be provided in order for your study to be reviewed. It may require that your protocol be presented in a specific order, and it may have template forms for subjects' consent.

In terms of general rules for protection of human subjects, safety, risk/benefits, and protection of particularly vulnerable populations such as children, the mentally ill, prisoners, and the elderly are the issues of concern. The proposal and consent form are reviewed to determine if the study is safe, if the benefits outweigh the risks, if risks are all identified for the potential subjects, and if special measures have been taken to protect vulnerable subjects, such as adapting the language of the consent form to their level of understanding, checking that the subject understands, or obtaining the consent of a caregiver or conservator if the participant is legally conserved or a minor. The reviewers also examine the consent form and the protocol to ensure congruity between the two documents. Exemption from having to obtain formal written consent from human subjects is a possibility if your study meets certain very specific criteria. Survey and educational studies may be exempt, as well as studies that examine preexisting samples of, for example, tissue or blood. You can ask the institution for its guidelines regarding exemption from obtaining human subjects' consent. If your study meets any of the exempted criteria, you can apply for exemption. The exemptions previously mentioned are in the federal guidelines. You can check on whether the institution uses the federal government exemption from human subjects' consent. Whatever guidelines an IRB uses should be made available to you. Human subjects approval may be required before the scientific merit is judged and approval is given to conduct the study. In other words, a study can have scientific merit but not be approved because of human subjects concerns and issues.

SCIENTIFIC MERIT REVIEW PROCESS

Scientific merit is judged in a number of ways. The reviewer or reviewers are usually given specific questions to ask about the proposal. Some organizations use checklists as a form of review; others rely upon the breadth and depth of knowledge of the reviewer to determine the scientific merit of a proposal. It is not an overgeneralization to point out that quantitative research proposals may be viewed as more "scientific" than qualitative proposals. But whether the research is quantitative or qualitative or both, the reviewer will look carefully at the proposal for evidence of its rigor. Is the methodology sound? Are the tools valid and reliable? Will new information be obtained? Is the sample size large enough to contribute to the body of knowledge? Is the investigator qualified to conduct the research? Are proper resources identified? Is the budget adequate? Are statistical measures sound?

QUALITATIVE ISSUES

Ethnographic participant observation without other forms of gathering data *may* qualify for an exemption from obtaining formal written consent from human subjects. There are, however, situations where you *must* apply for human subjects' consent. First, the situations that may qualify you for a human subjects exemption:

1. You will be observing a variety of staff or patients, and no one will be or can potentially be identified as part of your study. For example, you will observe while sitting in a lobby or a clinic where staff, patients, and families accumulate or pass through. A very early observation study as part of a focused ethnography that JR did involved observing psychiatric patients as they were being processed through admissions. The purpose was to understand the admissions process. Administration was particularly interested in learning if there were systems issues that made patients less likely to complete the admissions process. JR sat in the admis-

sions area, observing patients, families, and staff, but did not obtain consent from any of the participants. She did not know the patient identities and hence could not violate human consent guidelines. Though she did know the staff, no one was identified by name or position in her report to administration. First of all, it would have been almost impossible to get informed consent from the large number of patients, family, and staff in the area, and second, no privacy issues seemed to be violated. She did, however, obtain approval before doing the study from the person who was in charge of the admission area where observations took place.

2. You are using the participant-only method in your job as a staff member and collecting data covertly. We do not recommend this method of data collection, and IRBs usually not approve this type of study. Although this form of ethnography has been conducted, the implicit ethical problems discredit participant-only endeavors (see Chapter 2).

The key to deciding whether you need to complete a consent form and have human subjects review is an ethics and privacy concern. If you are observing sensitive procedures such as abortions, labor and delivery, electro-convulsive treatment (ECT), or other invasive procedures, you should get consent from the patient and staff subjects. Because these procedures may be sensitive for both staff and patients and invasive for the patient, you want to ensure that you have protected their rights by getting informed consent. Some subjects might not want an uninvolved observer reporting on what happens to them during these invasive procedures.

GETTING APPROVAL FROM THE IRB
FOR YOUR QUALITATIVE RESEARCH

This section describes issues specific to the processing of qualitative and ethnographic research. Nurses conducting purely qualitative and ethnographic research have difficulties getting approval from review boards. Part of the reason for this is the small number of traditional "scientific" staff who are knowledgeable about qualitative methodologies and analyses. The usual members of an IRB have never conducted qualitative research, so they may not understand the method and may believe that qualitative studies lack scientific rigor and are without replicability. It is up to you, the investigator, to highlight in your proposal for the nonqualitative researcher/reviewer those steps that will be taken to increase scientific rigor and clarity. As recommended by Morse (1991), having the formal support of an experienced ethnographer will add to your credibility in the eyes of review boards. In the chapter on writing the proposal, these issues are addressed in detail. In summary, remember these key points in your proposal:

- In your methodology section, give specific information regarding the actual steps in the conduct of ethnography, and specify what ethnography does for your study.

- Address the issues of reliability and validity. Nonqualitative researchers often view ethnographic research skeptically in relation to these issues.

- Be honest about the potential pitfalls of ethnographic research. Address them before the reviewer has a chance to think of them. Tell the reader how, despite the problems associated with ethnographic research, the methodology is the most effective way of answering the research question.

- Include your projected data analysis strategies. Remember, even in qualitative research, data analysis is outlined in the proposal. So tell the reader what the steps are in ethnographic analyses. If you are relating information in narratives to numbers, tell the reviewer about that process. Allow yourself some flexibility for conducting the actual analysis. If you are doing content analysis, explain that in detail. These strategies are not set in concrete: What you actually do in data analysis may vary somewhat from the plan projected in the proposal because of the nature of ethnographic research. But explain enough so that the reviewer understands the data analysis process for your specific study.

ACCESSING YOUR POPULATION/SITUATION

After successfully completing the formal review process, you are ready to contact the population projected as participants in your study. In ethnographic research, there are no specific guidelines to help you cross the barriers to your participants. Much depends on you and your skills in negotiating and forming relationships (Burgess, 1984b). Your knowledge of nursing may assist you in this process, but you must not assume that just because you are a nurse the barriers will be easily overcome.

Preston (1997) reported that he found it easier to gain access to his participants by approaching them as an anthropologist and not as a nurse. However, some situations are more difficult than others. Gordon (1987) studied a religious group whose members continually tried to convert him to their religious beliefs. Such groups may readily agree to the ethnographer's role in their group but at the price of total commitment and participation. As Kauffman (1994) learned, ethnicity and age represented a barrier to entry into one community. Cassell (1992), a woman, obtained admission to a predominantly male subculture of surgeons. She recognized the biases that may have been the consequence of the gender differences.

Entry to your population is a gradual process. A good example of that was our need to include other facilities, besides our own, in the data collection for our agitation study (Roper & Shapira, 1998, in review). We sought the assistance of a large private nursing home by first contacting the director of nurses and explaining the project to her. Once she had approved of the project, the study was reviewed by a formal IRB and approved. We then had to contact the director of nurses again to meet with staff to inform them about the study. Several meetings were held on all three tours to orient staff to the project. Then each nurse caregiver was approached individually for informed consent as a study participant. This total process took months!

Even though you have obtained institutional approval, barriers will still exist. In ethnographic participant observation, closeness to your subjects is required. This may frighten your subjects. Nursing staff may not like to be observed or may not allow you to observe those situations that you want to see. Participants may stop talking when you enter the room. These are probably more formidable barriers than you have ever encountered. You are a nurse, and yet you are not part of the culture or situation you want to study. Participants may assume that you are there to "spy" on them, even though you have told them differently. Or you are a nurse in the setting or situation, and you now want to observe others—staff you have worked with on a collegial basis. Initial hesitation on the part of nursing staff to allow you to conduct your study is to be expected.

These barriers can usually be overcome by "hanging in there." You may be tested as to whether you can be trusted with the knowledge and information that you gather as a result of your study. As indicated earlier in this chapter, you may want to observe particularly "sensitive" procedures or interactions, but the participants involved in these procedures may not want to be observed by an outsider. Do not assume that you will automatically be included in all events. Access may also depend on the role of the ethnographer. If you are more participant than observer, you will probably have access to most situations, perhaps to the detriment of observation.

Germain (1979) described in some detail the process she went through to gain access to the oncology unit staff and patients. She originally had wanted to observe a medical/surgical unit, but the hospital administrator directed her to the oncology unit because it had fewer physicians, fewer patients, and no students. But before she could even set foot on the unit, she had to get approval from the nursing supervisor and the medical director of the oncology unit, obtain a written legal contract between the university (her employer) and the hospital to protect the hospital from any problems arising from her research, and assure the facility of her professional license and personal liability insurance. She was instructed to wear a white lab coat and ID badge. After completing these steps, she was introduced to the head nurse of the oncology unit, who promptly put her on the time schedule as a staff nurse. The researcher had to clarify her role as researcher and as observer as well as participant. Ethnographic strategies seemed to work well, for eventually the director of nursing observed that the staff seemed to accept the researcher as one of their own.

Street (1992) was less clear about her process of gaining access. However, she did identify the gatekeepers of the institution as the nurse-researcher, the director of nursing (who later became sponsors of her study), the hospital research staff, and the medical/administrative staff. The one strategy that appeared to assist Street in her access to her participants was conducting an initial pilot study once she was in the facility. She began by enlisting the assistance of two staff to be participants in her pilot. She was gradually able to enlarge her contacts in the setting for the project.

Street (1992) summarized gaining access as a process that requires locating sponsors (staff who will support your study and introduce it to others), getting past gatekeepers, and then accessing the people at the field site (p. 121). These principles apply to most settings.

SUMMARY

Getting your foot in the door is generally a two-step process.

1. You first must get institutional approval through the formal mech- a- nisms of the setting. This process differs for each organization. Learn all you can about the procedures to facilitate approval of your study.

2. Then you must gain access to your special population or participants. Be- cause there are no standards for this step, you have to rely upon your ability to work effectively with people to negotiate and build trusting re- lationships.

6

NOW GO DO IT!

I wanted to live deep and suck out all the marrow of life.
Henry David Thoreau, *Walden* (1854;
cited in Sherwin, 1969, p. 44)

By now you have formulated a research question concerned with the ways a group of people behave and think. You want to learn about the everyday world of these participants and understand their views. The ethnographer goes into the field with the aim of discovery and becomes a human instrument who perceptively gathers information from people and events (Fetterman, 1989, p. 41) and then makes sense of what is seen by identifying patterns and formulating scientific explanations. Remember that you enter your place of study with an open mind to determine both consistencies and variations in patterns of behavior and knowledge. Data collection and analysis are done concurrently in a dialectic process as you strive to make sense of what you perceive (Agar, 1980, p. 9; Werner & Schoepfle, 1987, p. 23).

Ethnographic research permits an investigator to gain a broad and deep perspective of the group under study. But contained within this world are the complexities and ambiguities of real life. You will learn to cherish the potential "richness of contradictions" (Agar, 1980, p. 49) as the means to more fully understand the interactive processes and salient meanings of the people and culture. Through ethnographic activities, you are connected to individuals and events in a personal sense. Lofland (1971) described the types of closeness inherent in the ethnographic process. You are physically close as you interact face to face with group members over an extended period of time. A social closeness evolves as trust develops and confidences are shared with the investigator. And written descriptions of observations and analyses are detailed as you pay close attention to the patterns and variations of daily activities.

Though fieldwork is personal, it is not casual observation. Use of systematic methods channels subjective observations and conversations into data that can be analyzed objectively. Describing events in detail allows you to understand cultural behavior, or why people do what they do in a particular setting and at a particular time. The approach of ethnographic research incorporates a variety of techniques and a blending of strategies to capture this information, including participant observation, interviewing, and examination of available documents. In this chapter, we provide concrete methods to help answer the following questions: What do I do first? What methods do I use to observe? How do I talk to people? What and who should I observe? What other information should I collect? Can I trust my data? How do I document what I learn? How do I end my project?

WHAT DO I DO FIRST?
EXPLORATORY PARTICIPANT OBSERVATION

GAINING ENTRY

The first month or so of fieldwork is frightening and exciting. You are a stranger to the people of study; you don't know them, and they don't know you. But their world is open, waiting to be discovered. Accept that this period is unique for both you and the people you hope will become your teachers. As you begin to observe the setting, recognize that you, too, are being observed. People want to know who you are and what you plan to do. Present your project honestly and briefly; those who wish to know more will ask specific questions. For example, when JS introduced herself to staff nurses in the intensive care unit (ICU), she explained that she was interested in learning what it was like to care for agitated patients in that environment.

Wax (1971) described this period as a time of trying on roles that will allow you to conduct your research. During the introductory period in the ICU, JS soon realized that nurses had various ideas about what her role should be. One nurse hoped that her study of agitated patients would lead her to tell nursing administration to increase the staffing ratio of the unit. Another suggested that she speak to the doctors about changing the current medication policy for agitated patients. In response to these comments, she explained that the nurses were the experts and that she hoped to learn about those issues of most importance to them. A third wanted her to inform on nurses who were not following physicians' orders correctly. She clearly stated that she would not do this, as what she was told and what she observed would be considered confidential material. While you learn what people expect of you, there is a joint process of negotiation as you share with them what you are able to do. Just as you respect the members of the group you are studying, you must have a firm understanding of what you feel comfortable and ethical in reporting. The initial entry period is the time to clarify with yourself and others what your role will be.

Be prepared for *culture shock* (Brink & Saunders, 1976) or feelings of disorientation when you realize that you do not know how to respond and that you do not know the rules. This is especially notable when you are in a place far from home, away from family and friends, and do not have a good command of the language. One of our anthropology colleagues reads paperback novels, whereas another gets very cranky during this period. Keep track of these feelings by writing in your personal journal (to be described below). Not only will this diary serve as a coping mechanism, but you can also relate the early observations you make about the people and place to your reactions of loneliness, anxiety, or euphoria. Thus, you can identify any prejudices coloring your initial impressions of the study site. (See Jean Briggs's 1970 description of her loneliness and despair when working with an isolated group in Alaska.)

Working within your own culture and language may lessen the degree of confusion, but there is still an interval of feeling incompetent; it will pass as you become more accustomed to the surroundings. Another potential problem exists, however. If you study in a familiar setting, you already know many of the customs and norms, but there is a danger of missing important details that you take for granted. The entry period allows you to discover what assumptions you make unconsciously and helps you see things in a fresh way. When JS began exploratory observations in the evaluations and admissions area during a study of psychiatric patients with concurrent medical problems, she realized that she *expected* medical nurses to treat psychiatric patients "rudely." By acknowledging this bias early in the research process, she prevented invalid interpretations of the data collected during the remainder of the study (Agar, 1980, pp. 41-42). She also recognized that she had to purposefully avoid evaluating and judging what she saw during this early period. Once she was able to sit back and experience the environment without the usual nursing responsibilities, she was amazed at how much she learned about things she thought she already knew!

As you experience perceptions and feelings about the people and place, you begin to get a sense of where to focus. You are now ready to do a general survey.

GENERAL SURVEY

During the phase of exploratory participant observation, you first want to obtain the "big picture" of all the people and events in the group of study. Then, as you narrow the focus of inquiry while conducting more systematic data gathering, you can understand finer details within this larger perspective. Fetterman (1989) called this the "big net approach" (pp. 42-43).

First take a census of the setting (Pelto & Pelto, 1978). Find out who are the members of the group. For example, if you are conducting a community study, determine how many people live in the area. If you are visiting people in their homes, note material goods such as televisions, computers, and refrigerators. If you are working with a homeless population, identify items they consider essential for survival (Pelto & Pelto, 1978). In a hospital, record the number of patients seen in 1 year and the distribution of medical and nursing staff members. For a contained area, such as a nursing home or hospital unit, describe the number of rooms, patients per room, and nursing staff. You may want to draw a map of the spatial arrangement: location of the nursing station, or size of the patients' dining room in comparison to the physicians' eating area. Locate where major social action and interaction takes place. One anthropologist who studied an acute psychiatric ward asked all staff members to draw a map of the same space; she then compared their different perspectives through these drawings. Interestingly, in the social worker's picture, the telephone was prominently displayed (Rhodes, 1991).

This general survey also includes an overview of the different cliques or mini-group memberships. When you are ready to do more systematic data collection, make sure you get input from all appropriate people. When you latch on to one person early, that world is open to you, but you may unwittingly cut yourself off from knowledge of other groups. Attend carefully to who first approaches you. When Michael Agar (1980) conducted an ethnography of heroin addicts, he found that he was often first approached by "stranger-handlers" trying to figure out who he was and then reporting back to the group (p. 85). Agar also cautioned about "deviants," people on the outside of a group who hope to increase their status by association with you (p 86). Though it is important to understand the perspectives of all members of the society, make sure to establish their positions to determine if they represent majority or minority views.

During this period of introduction, concentrate on listening. If you ask too many questions before people are used to you, they may feel threatened. It has been our experience that people will eventually want to talk with you, particularly if you are genuinely interested in them as individuals and in what they do. Everyone likes a good listener. You may also try to reciprocate whenever possible. Anthropologists in the field share food and transportation. JS helps nurses in the ICU as they give bed baths and change linen.

This is an exciting period because you gain acceptance into the group and confidence in your ability to communicate. You learn a great deal during this initial stage of participant observation as you discern patterns of behavior and domains appropriate for more intensive and systematic observations during the next phase of your ethnographic project. We now describe specific participant observation strategies used in ethnographic research.

WHAT IS THE PROCESS OF ETHNOGRAPHIC
PARTICIPANT OBSERVATION?

Ethnographic participant observation is the "interweaving of looking, listening, and asking" (Lofland, 1971, p. 109) to gain understanding about people, events, and cultural systems. There are two principal purposes of participant observation. You watch an activity, find it intriguing, and then ask a group member to explain its meaning to you. Or participating in and observing activities can be used to test the results of what you have been told during formal and informal interviews. While conducting ethnographic research, you strategically link what you see with what you are told. Relying on personal observations alone can be misleading, as perceptions are filtered through one's cultural background, previous knowledge, and systems of meaning. Remember, the aim is to observe and understand the world from the view of its members and then apply your own interpretations and explanations. This interplay of emic and etic perspectives permits the deep and rich insights associated with ethnography and is accomplished by ethnographic observational strategies.

OBSERVATIONAL APPROACHES IN ETHNOGRAPHY

The types of observations made change as the project evolves. Spradley (1980) specified descriptive, focused, and selective observational approaches. *Descriptive* observations are made during the general survey in the exploratory phase of the study. These observations are not systematic; the objective is to become aware of the variety of events that occur during a usual day and to note topics to be studied in more depth later. The records of these initial observations in field notes may appear obsessively detailed, as you do not yet know what is going to prove significant. For example, in JS's study in the triage area of the evaluations department, she first sat in the chairs in the waiting area and tried to describe everything she saw: the patients waiting for care, the procedure of evaluation, the comments made by family members, and actions of the triage nurses.

Following these early encounters, observations become more *focused* and systematic. Decisions are made to attend to some aspects of the environment and ignore others. In the study described above, the question of when a "person" entering the evaluations area became a "patient" proved meaningful; thus, JS spent several days identifying the various steps of the screening process.

Selective observations come last. Focus is sharpened as you concentrate on specific attributes of activities. Checklists may be developed to capture behaviors and events systematically. For example, when patients were examined in the emergency room, JS used a grid to register their behaviors (grimacing, smiling, talking, moving, etc.) and the actions of the professional staff (smiling, talking, touching, time spent with patient, etc.).

In whatever way you decide to focus your observations, it is necessary to have a strategy to collect useful information. It may be as general as newspaper reporters' "five W's and an H"—who, what, when, where, why, and how (Agar, 1980, p. 92)—or may be more specific. Whiting and Whiting (1973) described four "genres of observation." First, record the *places, stages, and sets* where an event occurs. A place might be the specific hospital, a stage might be the particular ward, and various possible sets might be the patient's bed, a nursing station, a break room, or a family waiting room. Note any *objects* used in the event, such as leather restraints to control an agitated patient. Identify the *persons or actors* in the set, either all of them or selected individuals. Finally, describe the *activities or performances* you observe; remember to validate your interpretations with those of group members.

Often, the event observed includes verbal communication between individuals. In his "ethnography of speaking," Hymes (1972) identified features that influence patterns of speech behavior. He coined the mnemonic *SPEAKING* (Setting, Participants, Ends, Act, Key, Instrumentality, Norms, Genre) as a reminder of observations to make. *Setting* is represented by two domains: physical and psychological. Physical setting indicates when and where the speech event occurs; note the architectural space and arrangement of the speakers. To determine psychological setting, describe the mood that participants bring to the event. Describe the *participants* and see if you can identify the leaders. *Ends* are the expected outcomes or goals of a speech event. Analyze both the (emic) belief systems of the participants and your (etic) perspective of the purpose of the activity. Focusing on the *act* sequence reveals how the content of the encounter is ordered: What happens first? What is the response of one person to the actions of another? The *key* of the event is the emotional tone of the participants that develops during the interaction. Try to evaluate the affect and mood of the setting. *Instrumentality* includes the dialect or linguistic variety used by the community during the observed event. For example, do adolescents in the group use words in the same way as adults? Does joking occur? What are the uses of silence? By attending to the *norms* of the group, one can compare ideal and actual behavior. Perhaps nurses in a setting have told you that they have a balanced collegial relationship with the physicians in their unit. But you observe during rounds that physicians speak more often and interrupt nursing staff frequently. This discrepancy would be interesting to investigate further. The *genre* of an event tells the participants how to behave in the situation. We speak and act differently in a seminar on nursing research methods than we do at a party. Note systematic patterns that occur within different genres. This method of analyzing events is complex but yields a great deal of information about the participants. Anderson (1996) used these strategies to explore the interactional dynamics among young women in juvenile detention as they participated in group discussions, individual interviews, and daily activities. Verbal and nonverbal behaviors of the participants were observed and analyzed.

Regardless of the system chosen to observe discrete events and interactions, one key strategy is to be open to the surroundings. Use all your senses while observing: Is it cold in the room, is there an unpleasant odor, are the magazines in the waiting room recent or outdated? Another strategy is to be systematic and concrete. There is a trend in ethnographic research toward quantifying data whenever possible (Bernard, 1994; Johnson & Johnson, 1990); this allows readers to situate your findings within a larger perspective and permits them to agree or disagree with your interpretation of the situation. For example, we find it more helpful to know that "18 out of 20 people in the waiting room were women" than to know that "most of the people waiting were women." The waiting room becomes more visible to the reader when more information is known. Finally, always check your interpretations of the observed actions with members of the group by asking questions through casual conversations or formal interviews.

HOW DO I TALK TO PEOPLE?
ETHNOGRAPHIC INTERVIEWING

As you observe activities of individuals and group events, many questions will come to mind. The aim of ethnography is to discover the answers from the members of the cultural group and also to interpret what you see from your own perspective. Group, informal, and formal interviewing procedures are used to elicit these explanations.

Whether speaking casually to one person in a public space or asking specific questions in a private room, always use a respectful approach. Consider cultural values by learning what is appropriate in the setting, including proper dress. Just as you wait for an invitation before entering another's home, obtain permission before intruding into an area used by group members. For example, JR asked permission to attend team meetings, and JS did not go behind the desk of the nurses' station in the ICU until invited. People are helping you when they answer questions. Respect their time. Adapt your schedule to one that works best for them, and be willing to cancel your meeting at any time. When we went to speak with nurses at an agreed-upon time and found them busy with patient care, we came back later. Also be aware of participants' moods; they may have agreed to speak with you on a certain date, but they may not really feel like talking when the day arrives. Recognize that people may get tired of answering questions, particularly about events you observe together.

Remember to let participants talk—the goal is to learn what *they* believe and know. Be nonjudgmental; even if you do not agree with what someone tells you, try to understand his or her point of view. Learn to use silence; after asking a question, provide enough time for reflection. Finally, how you shape the questions influences responses (Pelto & Pelto, 1978). For example, if you ask only about negative things (i.e., stigma of psychiatric patients or stress in the ICU), people will tell you only about negative things. Be open to learn from people during group, informal, and formal interviews.

GROUP INTERVIEWS

Interviewing a group of people at the same time may be done during the beginning stages of your project. Just as a general survey gives a sense of the physical environment, a group interview alerts you to the variation in ideas and concepts present among the population. This techniques is most productive when focused on topics that are reasonably public and not sensitive or embarrassing (Lofland, 1971, p. 88). Being part of a group allows people time to reflect upon and recall their experiences; they do not feel as pressured to respond as do participants in private interviews. Comments of others may trigger memories or incidents that enrich the discussion. And when people disagree, you quickly obtain an awareness of possible contrasting perspectives about specific issues. We conducted a series of group interviews with nursing staff after completing exploratory participant observation during our pilot ethnography of agitation among patients with dementia. We used information we learned from these nurses to formulate focused interview questions during a later stage of the study. We realized the importance of having both of us attend these group interviews; while one asked questions, the other observed the interactional dynamics of the group.

INFORMAL INTERVIEWS

Asking questions about observed events and interactions immediately after they occur allows you to discover the meanings of these activities to group members. Informal or casual conversation is a way to identify the range and consensus of beliefs about a specific event (Fetterman, 1989). By requesting explanations, the ethnographer places discrete observations into the larger cultural context. Informal interviews are not prearranged but follow what is happening in the "here and now" (Agar, 1980, p. 90). Rather than following a list of specific topics, you develop a general approach for asking questions. Let the research participant take the lead and describe what is significant in the situation while you look interested in what you are told. Ask questions about issues that are puzzling or lead to a specific area of interest. For example, after talking casually to patients waiting to be evaluated in the admissions area, JS asked if they had been waiting long. Informal interviewing can occur anywhere—in the break room, at the nurses' station, in the parking lot. One of the primary values of these natural conversations is the immediate feedback obtained after observing a situation, while the information is still fresh and easily recalled. Finally, by asking interested questions and listening carefully to the responses, you develop and maintain a positive rapport with your informants.

FORMAL INTERVIEWS

Formal or focused interviews use a systematic approach to obtain desired information from participants. The specific questions asked are developed after you have spent some time with the group and have a general understanding of the setting and patterns of interaction among participants. This allows you to pose questions that reflect the participants' worldview and not merely what you believe.

Design an interview guide containing a list of topics of interest to you. The questions are open-ended as you gently guide the direction of the conversation. Start with general questions (i.e., "What is it like for you to be a nurse?"), and then ask for more detailed material as the interview proceeds (i.e., "What patients are most difficult for you?"). Use probes to elicit detailed information (i.e., "You mentioned that your mother was a nurse— could you tell me more about that?"). You may want to purposefully make a claim to see if you are contradicted (Agar, 1980). For example, if you have noticed that nurses seem to work separately rather than together, you might state, "The nurses seem to work together and share their assignments—is that so?" We also find it illuminating to ask informants how others act, believe, or feel. During our agitation study (Roper & Shapira, 1999), we received quite different answers when we asked these two questions: "What do you do when a patient becomes agitated?" and "What do other nurses do?"

In addition to asking directed questions, note the effect of the questions on the participant. Attend to nonverbal cues, such as speed of speaking, presence or absence of eye contact, and emotional outbursts of laughter or tears. A shift in the conversation may indicate an issue of particular significance for the individual that deserves following. Be aware of the balance between probing for deep feelings and beliefs and being intrusive. When we asked caregiver spouses of AD patients about their feelings related to caregiving, every person cried at some point during the interview but did not want to stop the discussion. Good listeners elicit meaningful thoughts and feelings from participants who are willing to share their thoughts and experiences. As is discussed in the next chapter, all participants must be informed of the nature of the questions before the interview begins and allowed to stop whenever they desire.

Most formal interviews are tape recorded so that complete attention can be given to what is being said. It is useful to make a separate written interview guide for each interviewee. Notes can be written of key words of the directed conversation and what is left to be covered. Prepare for the interview by checking the equipment before the informant arrives. If you have agreed to pay the participants for their time, make sure you have the correct amount of money and a receipt slip available. Finally, leave enough time for a postinterview, and allow people to ask you questions about yourself or the project.

Witnessing and participating in events and activities and then asking questions of group members are two components of the process of ethnography. You, as the researcher, interpret what you have learned through these observations and interviews. You determine what to watch, whom to question, and how to participate in group functions. Because this can be a subjective process, you must take care to represent the full range of activities in the setting and to learn as much as possible from individuals with varied points of view by using sampling techniques in the research process.

WHOM DO I QUESTION AND
WHAT DO I OBSERVE? SAMPLING

During ethnography, the researcher links the activities of looking, listening, and asking questions to learn from group members. The two primary sources of information are people and events. Remember, one of your goals is to understand the world through its members by discovering what is important in their eyes and what meaning specific behaviors have for them.

KEY INFORMANTS

When first entering the study site, you are introduced to most of the people in the setting. Some seem interested in speaking with you, whereas others pretty much ignore your presence. Once you have talked to several people, the "well-informed informant" emerges (Werner & Schoepfle, 1987, p. 184). The term *informant* was coined by anthropologists to describe a person willing to help by explaining the customs and beliefs of the identified cultural group. Often this person spoke the language of the anthropologist. The word *informant* has come under scrutiny recently; in Western culture, it has a negative connotation as someone who informs or tells on others. Also, social scientists are now consciously aware of the interactive nature of ethnography and wish to acknowledge the significant relationship between the investigator-as-student and informant-as-teacher. Thus, informants are called *key actors* (Fetterman, 1989), *respondents* (Lofland, 1971), and *consultants* (Werner & Schoepfle, 1987). In this chapter, we respectfully label as *key informants* those people willing to share time and knowledge to teach us about their lives.

Key informants have several notable characteristics. They are usually from the mainstream of the group and can relate the history of the group to what is happening today. Key informants are broadly knowledgeable but can also objectively reflect on their general culture and processes outside of their personal experiences. When conducting a focused ethnographic study, choose key informants who have directly experienced the phenomenon of interest. Often your key informants are "culture brokers" (Fetterman, 1989, p. 58) who can explain things from different perspectives. For example, in JS's study of psychiatric patients with concurrent medical problems, one key informant was an office assistant who had medical and psychiatric diagnoses; he was able to reflect on his experiences as both patient and employee serving other patients.

Several years ago, we were key informants in a study conducted by an undergraduate anthropology student. She was exploring the different roles women use in the workplace. We both greatly enjoyed the experience, as the student was a good listener and asked insightful questions. We were conscious of differing layers of our responses: Our explanations were derived from both personal experiences and our shared or cultural understandings of the institution in which we worked. Key informants are used to validate information that you get from other sources, such as observations you make or statements from other group members. They also provide feedback when you are ready to make hypotheses about what is happening or why things occur. Although key informants can be extremely helpful to you in understanding events and people, do not rely solely on them to provide the information you need. Choose other representatives to obtain their perspectives of the situation too.

SAMPLES OF PEOPLE

To have confidence in the results of your study, you must convince yourself and your readers that you have observed and spoken with a variety of members of the group. How you select these representatives depends upon your particular study design and the availability of potential participants. The most common types of samples used in ethnographic research are snowball samples, purposeful selection, solicited participants, and the total population of group members. Probability sampling (i.e., random or stratified) techniques may prove helpful in some study designs.

During the initial phase of exploratory participant observation, you can identify participants who suggest others in their social group to include in your study. This is described variously as a *snowball, opportunist,* or *nominated sample* (Agar, 1980; Brink & Wood, 1994; Morse, 1989). Each individual interested in your study helps select another participant by either directly recruiting the new subject for the investigator or permitting the investigator to name him or her as a reference. If you have selected appropriate individuals who are knowledgeable about their cultural group, they can recommend others who will also provide competent information. Because someone they know and trust introduces them to you, potential participants are more likely to speak with you. This strategy is particularly useful when studying vulnerable individuals who may not wish to be identified, such as persons with AIDS, families of suicides, or people with issues of substance abuse. Morse (1989) pointed out, however, that you must choose participants who truly want to help, as you give them the control over recruiting subjects.

A *purposeful, theoretical,* or *judgmental sample* (Agar, 1980; Fetterman, 1989; Glaser & Strauss, 1967) includes people selected because they are specialists or experts in some area of interest to you as defined by your research questions. You choose people to interview in a deliberate way to obtain data to compare with what you have already discov-

ered. By checking similarities and differences of the information provided and seeking out people with wide ranges of experiences, you
attain a more complete understanding of phenomena and concepts.
Again, experts are identified during the general survey at the beginning
of the project and after initial interviews with study participants. When
a specific question is answered to your satisfaction and you are no longer
learning new material, obtain a different sample of people purposefully
selected to reveal additional data.

Solicited samples (Agar, 1980) are used when the researcher may not
know potential participants. Individuals are often recruited from organized groups. McGarrahan (1994) became a member of a nurses' spe-
cialty organization (Association of Nurses in AIDS Care) and requested
participation from fellow members when she studied the experiences of
nurses who cared for AIDS patients. Recognize, however, that people
who join organizations may have different experiences from those who
do not use these resources (Morse, 1989). Variation in sample selection
is increased when you extend your recruitment to a more general audience through advertisements in newspapers, on the radio, and on televi-
sion (Morse, 1989).

When studying a group of people who live or work in a specific area,
research interaction with the *total population* is possible. Single house-
holds or all patients and staff on a single unit are examples. JR approached all of the nursing staff working in the psychiatric intensive
care unit for her study on restraints and seclusion. She found that some
individuals were better able to enlighten her but that inviting all to participate allowed her greater access during the periods of observation.

Probability sampling techniques can be used in ethnographic research
if the population characteristics are known. *Random sampling* occurs
after the completion of a general survey that documents the variation
that is present among the total population in the setting. For example,
you might obtain a list of all the nurses who work in a hospital, or all patients seen in a particular clinic, and then randomly select people from
this pool for intensive study. Note that people are not chosen because of
their special knowledge or expertise and thus may not be key informants
of the cultural system. A *stratified* or *quota sample* (Agar, 1980; Brink &
Wood, 1994) is based on percentages of characteristics discovered in the
general survey to ensure heterogeneity of the sample. For example, the

background literature reviewed for our agitation study (Roper & Shapira, 1999) revealed a potential difference in experiences of caregivers based on demographic variables. We thus sampled nurse caregivers who worked in both private and public nursing homes and male and female spouse caregivers. Caution must be used with this strategy, however, as decisions may be made to include people with characteristics that do not truly reflect the variations of the phenomenon being studied. Morse (1989) questioned the threat to validity when using a sampling procedure based on the quota system: Key informants may be excluded because their subgroup has already been interviewed.

Regardless of the type of sample used, keep careful and detailed field notes describing the reasoning used as people are selected for your study. Discuss who agreed to talk with you and who refused. Reflect in your field notes if you believe you obtained input from all layers of the group; if not, state how this might affect the interpretations made in your written report. In particular, the ongoing relationship with key informants influences the direction of the project, and your personal feelings about these essential individuals might be noted in the personal diary.

SAMPLES OF EVENTS

When in the field, you cannot be everywhere at once and observe all that occurs. Just as you make decisions about certain people to interview, you also choose activities and events to monitor. The general survey conducted during the exploratory phase of the project alerts you to the events of most salience to the members of the group: What do people talk about, where do most people go, when are critical ceremonies and meetings held? Agar (1980) suggested three ways to learn about happenings in the community. First, of course, you hope to directly observe the event yourself. Second, you can record what people recall about an event that you did not witness. Many days JS would enter the evaluation area to have a nurse tell her, "You should have been here last night. We had a patient who . . . ." (She became convinced that the "good" things only happened when she was home sleeping!) In this case, ask several people involved with the event to describe what they recall; you can then test some assumptions you have about the phenomenon. Finally, you can create hypothetical cases to gauge the degree of agreement among people. For example, ask, "What would happen if . . . ?"

These techniques allow you to understand different events even when you are not physically present.

In addition to observing significant events as they occur, random spot checks of what people do throughout the day alerts you to habitual patterns of behavior and allows you to determine the frequency of "significant" events. By sampling a sufficiently large number of representative acts, you will be able to approximate the percentage of time people spend doing an activity or a specific behavior and get a firm sense of normal daily routine (Bernard, 1994; Gross, 1984; Johnson, 1978). JS has incorporated this strategy in her study exploring the impact of agitated patient behaviors on the patterns of ICU nurses' caregiving. Random spot observations will be made on the 12 patient beds in the intensive care unit. These data will be collected 5 days each week; 70% of the observations will occur from 7 a.m. to 7 p.m., and 30% will occur from 7 p.m. to 7 a.m. and on the weekends. On each of these days, six times of the day will be randomly selected. The order of bed observation will also be randomly selected. Conducting six observations per day for 5 days per week yields 1,080 observations in 9 months. These observations will be recorded on an observation checklist that will be finalized after the initial phase of exploratory participant observation. As can be seen from this design, the normal patterns and activities of the ICU as well as the more infrequent and unusual episodes of agitation can be observed. Thus, these sampling methods help you decide who and what should be studied in your ethnographic project. In addition to participant observation and interviewing techniques, ethnographic methods include supplementary data sources to describe relevant characteristics of the culture or group.

WHAT OTHER TYPES OF
INFORMATION DO I COLLECT?
SUPPLEMENTARY SOURCES OF INFORMATION

Because the process of ethnography is a holistic appraisal of the lifeways of a population or phenomenon of interest, knowledge about past events and changes over time helps you situate and understand the present (Germain, 1986). Relevant information may be included in written documents such as patient records, policies and procedures, patient educational materials, and newspaper articles. Data found in written archives or spoken life histories of participants reveal historical underpinnings of current events. For example, JS uncovered an unpublished history of the hospital where she conducts research, complete with black-and-white photographs, that outlined the original aims of the institution. Cultural artifacts or previous technological methods may also prove interesting. JR collected examples of various types of soft and leather restraints while conducting her ethnography. Finally, some ethnographers use close-ended questionnaires or inventories to collect standardized information from participants. However, because the intent of ethnography is to discover the meaning of events from the perspective of group members, reliance on information developed solely from "outsider" assumptions is limited in this type of research (Germain, 1993, p. 254). Thus, the three methods of ethnography—participant observation, interviewing, and consulting additional sources of information —combine to capture rich and essential patterns of participant behavior and beliefs. In addition, triangulation of these three types of data helps support claims that your methods and conclusions have validity and reliability, which are desired aims of all research.

VALIDITY AND RELIABILITY

Validity refers to the accuracy of the methods used to collect and analyze information collected during research (Bernard, 1994, p. 38). Validity is a major strength of the ethnographic process if the results reflect the reality and meanings of the group studied (LeCompte & Goetz, 1982). Remember that the goal of this research strategy is to study how people think and act in their natural setting. Because the investigator depends upon others to share their "truth," specific steps must be taken to increase confidence in the results.

The process of selecting events to observe and informants to question has been discussed above under sampling procedures and includes first conducting a general survey to identify the variation in people and activities. Describe the strategies used to obtain information from people knowledgeable about your research topic. Informants may respond with what they believe is the "correct" answer or may unconsciously present their group members in a positive light. Construct open-ended questions framed in neutral language, and ask the same questions several times, in different ways, over the course of the fieldwork. Spending a long period of time with participants increases the opportunity to assess the accuracy of both informants' statements and your own interpretations.

Validity of a research design is increased by designing multiple procedures to collect data on the same content (Brink, 1989b, p. 159), and ethnography, by definition, triangulates information from the three activities of participant observation, interviewing, and examination of supplementary data sources. What is learned from one method is checked against other sources. In her ICU study, JS observes agitated patient behaviors as they occur and concurrently interviews nursing staff about their beliefs and feelings of caring for agitated patients. In addition, she uses available written records of medications given and physical restraints applied to patients to validate what she observes and what she is told.

Reliability means that methods of collecting data are consistent, stable, and repeatable (Brink & Wood, 1994, p. 170). Constraints on reliability in participant observation studies occur because the research is conducted in naturalistic settings where variables are purposefully not controlled. Rather than viewing inconsistencies as problems with reliability, one can see conflicting perspectives as reflecting what actually happens in the real world (Jorgensen, 1989, p. 36). Reliability of both informants' statements, and the investigator's accuracy in collecting and recording data is taken into account (Brink, 1989b).

As with validity, reliability in ethnographic research is enhanced because the investigator has the opportunity to observe many events and to interview people multiple times during the extended period of data collection. The use of methods to collect systematic information allows confirmation of findings from several informants and thus increases confidence that cultural members view phenomena similarly (LeCompte & Goetz, 1982). Scrupulous attention to recording concrete and objective descriptions of events and verbatim accounts of conversations and interviews in field notes allows others to substantiate your interpretations. We turn now to a discussion of ways to record what you learn from participants, events, the setting, and yourself while conducting research.

TABLE 6.1	Excerpt From Notebook
The nurse approached the patient without introducing himself. He pulled the covers down. He gave the patient a shot. He did not speak or smile during the interaction.	*Seems unsympathetic to this patient. Does this nurse always act like this? How does this behavior compare with that of other nurses in the setting?*

HOW DO I DOCUMENT
WHAT I LEARN? FIELD NOTES

From the moment you begin your research experience, you will want to document your observations, conversations, feelings, and interpretations in field notes. The raw data in these recordings are then used for formal analysis (Agar, 1980, p. 112). Write things down; do not count on memory when faced with a barrage of new sights, people, and impressions. But when and how to document these findings presents challenges when conducting ethnography. If you are constantly sitting in a corner with your nose in a notebook, there is a danger of missing out on important activities. Yet if you delay until the end of the day you may not remember everything that happened. Also, if you wait too long, you may situate your immediate impressions in a preexisting category and thus miss new insights. Researchers develop their own styles of writing field notes. We offer suggestions that have been useful for us, but you will need to find a strategy that works best for you.

PARTIAL FIELD NOTES

First, cultivate the habit of remembering what you observe and hear. Make mental notes (Lofland, 1971, p. 102) so that later you will be able to put down on paper what is observed. These mental notes are used at times when it is inappropriate to take written notes—for example, when having a conversation with one person. Sometimes you can inconspicuously jot down little phrases, quotes, or key words that will later serve as cues when you are writing up notes at the end of the day (Lofland,

1971). JS keeps a small notebook in her pocket to capture these quick observations and rushes to a nearby bathroom to complete her writings.

COMPLETE FIELD NOTES

Full field notes consist of various types of material: a running description of observed events and people; conversations with and among people; your interpretations, analyses, and thoughts for further questions; and personal feelings about your experience. Like other investigators, we find that keeping two separate notebooks allows us to keep track of these different aspects of the project (Agar, 1980; Johnson & Johnson, 1990; Werner & Schoepfle, 1987).

There are various methods of documenting material in field notes; one technique used by JS is presented in this chapter. In the notebook describing your observations and conversations, divide each page in half lengthwise. On the left-hand side, write down the events as they occur; be concrete and do not summarize in these running notes. The goal is to capture behaviors and conversations. Strauss and Corbin (1990) suggested the following notation to document conversations: Place *exact recall* in quotation marks ("I don't mind waiting to see the doctor"); use apostrophes when *paraphrasing* ('It doesn't bother him to wait to see a doctor'); and when you have *fair recall* but not a direct quotation, do not use any marks (he said he would wait). On the right-hand side, there is space for analytic ideas, inferences, and perceptions of patterns and concepts (Lofland, 1971). You can also jot down additional questions to ask after reviewing these notes. Table 6.1 provides an example of a notation JS made in her notebook; concrete observations are on the left-hand side and comments on the right-hand side of the page. Photographs, pictures drawn by members of the group, and notices of meetings or parties can also be included in this notebook and can be pasted into it in chronological order.

A second notebook becomes a diary that focuses on your reactions to the people around you, the setting, and your feelings and emotions. These are personal and intimate notes to yourself and can be used to evaluate your response to specific observations and interviews. Anything that can affect your "emotional and intellectual balance" (Werner & Schoepfle, 1987, p. 274) should be recorded in this personal diary.

SYSTEMATIC DATA COLLECTION

Eventually you will identify from your notebooks salient categories and behavior patterns of interest to your study. Forms and checklists make data collection easier and serve as reminders of what to observe or ask. It is important to structure these observation guidelines after spending enough time in the field to learn what is important to the people of the group. These forms can be modified as new information becomes available. Systematic data are also obtained from written documents, such as staffing assignments, reports of medication errors, days spent in the hospital, and number of appointments missed. JS collected the number of minutes patient waited in the evaluations area before being discharged, compared waiting times of patients with different diagnoses, and then used this information to supplement her observations and interviews with patients and staff members.

COMMITMENT TO FIELD NOTES

Participant observation cannot be accomplished without complete and current field notes. Although it is more fun to be where the action is, you must be willing to reserve the time to transcribe your observations and thoughts to paper for ongoing and future analysis. Write promptly—within 24 hours of the observation if possible. It is better to spend fewer hours in the field if that allows you to keep up with your field notes. We find it easiest to transcribe the notes directly into a word-processing program. If you get in the habit of spending time daily with your field notes, written descriptions will have depth and color that will add to the final manuscript. Be sure to make copies of field notes and computer diskettes, and keep them in separate places: JR kept one copy in her car, one at home, and one at work. The notes you make about others are confidential and must be protected. We both assigned numbers to individual staff members that we interviewed and kept the coding sheet hidden during our research projects. In a small setting, people can be identified by the comments you record; aggregate the information so that specific individuals are not recognized.

Field notes are the records of your research activities. Like the general survey, they start unfocused and become more systematic as you choose target areas of interest. But in the process of selecting specific pathways of inquiry, alternative roads are ignored. Thus, you need to consciously use the sampling procedures previously described to decide whom to question and what to observe.

HELPFUL EQUIPMENT

You can use *pen and paper* to record field notes, information from interviews, and layouts of the physical setting. They are easy and inexpensive and do not require electricity. They are also unobtrusive and familiar to most people. When taking notes, however, it is hard to maintain eye contact during a face-to-face interview, and you miss events when looking down to write. Also, if you plan to use computer programs in analyzing the information, these handwritten notes must be transcribed into a compatible word-processing program.

Computers, particularly portable laptop models, save time, as notes can be recorded directly into them and merged with other data for analysis. But you need space and a power source to set them up, and you cannot move quickly to events as they occur. We find that taking field notes with pen and paper and then transcribing them within 24 hours into the computer is the most efficient strategy.

Tape recorders permit you to make eye contact, listen, and formulate additional questions during long interviews and conversations. Make sure to jot down a few key phrases in case there is an equipment malfunction during a critical session. You can also listen to the tapes and hear nuances in voices and significant pauses that contribute insight to the words themselves. Unfortunately, transferring audio recordings onto paper is labor intensive and expensive; the transcriptions must be double-checked for accuracy. To cut down on the time required, it is possible to transcribe the most relevant sections first and return to the remainder of the tape if the information is needed. JS bought a dictating machine that allows her to control the speed of the recording with her foot while typing; though helpful, each hour of tape still takes at least 2 hours to transcribe. In medical settings, special permission and consent are required before taping interviews. Also, some people are particularly shy around recording devices. Sometimes participants wait to bring up sensitive and salient material until the tape recorder is turned off; write a few of these phrases down, and fill in what you remember as soon as possible.

Photographs create a permanent picture of the setting and allow your audience to visually share your experience (Fetterman, 1989). They also remind you of specific details when writing your report. It is difficult to get authorization to take pictures in health care settings, as it is impossible to obtain written permission from all individuals who appear in the pictures. Hand-drawn pictures may serve as a substitute.

Videotaping "provides the observer with the ability to stop time" (Fetterman, 1989, p. 85). You can tape an event and watch it over and over to discover patterns in behavior and speech. Video cameras are generally unobtrusive, especially when placed away from participants' direct line of view. These devices capture what goes on naturally in the setting without the presence of a human investigator. Proctor and colleagues (1996) set up video cameras in a trauma unit and recorded the actions and verbalizations of comfort made by nurses. Note that the focus of this (nonethnographic, participant-only) study clearly occurred within a confined space that could be documented by the camera; events happening outside of this range could not be analyzed.

In sum, the process of ethnography involves an intricate relationship between the investigator and the people of the community. By specifying in field notes exactly how data were collected, the nature of your interactions with participants, and personal feelings while conducting the research, you can evaluate how this association influenced the results. We discuss these issues in more depth in Chapter 8.

HOW DO I END MY PROJECT?
CONCLUDING THE RESEARCH

There are several reasons to end a project. The most satisfying conclusion is to stay in the field until all the information needed to answer the research questions is obtained. Most investigators, however, have a limited amount of time designated for data collection; they know the approximate date of departure when beginning their study. Some ethnographers continue to visit research sites for many years after their initial studies, whereas others never return. Regardless of the duration of the relationship with the participants, specific steps taken by investigators assist in a smooth transition for all concerned.

As the time of departure nears, remind participants when you will leave. Feelings of ambivalence are to be expected. The relief of completing intensive data collection competes with a sense of sadness about leaving people with whom you have spent so much time. A public ceremony might be appropriate, or small gifts for close informants. When we concluded our agitation study in one nursing home, we brought pizzas for all staff members to thank them for helping us. Another site asked us to share our findings with the nurses. Leaving the site of data collection is not the end of the project. Some say this is when the real work begins, as you complete the analysis of data and write a final report!

SUMMARY

In this chapter, we described methods used to discover patterns in the activities and meanings of a group of people. The specific ethnographic methods of participant observation, interviewing, and collection of supplemental information were identified. The following are important points to remember:

- Obtain a general survey of the setting and participants during the initial phase of the study. Situate the information learned during focused observations and interviews within this larger perspective.

- Select events to observe and informants to question deliberately. Be prepared to explain how these decisions were made.

- Be committed to your field notes. Keep concrete and detailed descriptions of your observations and personal feelings.

- Be open, respectful, and nonjudgmental in all interactions with group participants. Value what they teach you about their world.

7

WHAT TO DO
WITH ALL THE DATA!

Numerous researchers have indicated that data does not speak for
itself.

R. G. Burgess, *In the Field* (1984b, p. 236)

Data analysis is the focus of this chapter. Ethnographers collect great
quantities of material to discover what people believe and how
they behave in everyday situations. This information is primarily con-
veyed in written words compiled from transcribed interviews of research participants, field notes of participant observation activities, and
descriptions of relevant documents. The purpose of ethnographic analysis is to organize the data and then make sense of what you have learned
during the research experience. The written material is first categorized
into meaningful pieces, which are then examined for patterns that explain the phenomena of interest. The analysis progresses to more abstract generalizations as you reveal, explain, and interpret how people
behave in everyday situations.

Data analysis is a challenging subject to explain. Only since the 1980s
has ethnographic analysis received some clarification in the qualitative
literature, and it remains uncommon for ethnographic reports to detail

their strategies for data analysis. Recently, some researchers (Burgess, 1984a; Fetterman, 1989; Miles & Huberman, 1994; Morse & Field, 1995) have devoted texts and chapters to specific guidelines for ethnographic analysis. None of the guidelines are exactly alike, but they do have some shared characteristics. They all agree that analysis is time consuming, is driven by the data, begins in the field while data are being collected, and requires specific methodological strategies to verify data and validate conclusions reached by the ethnographer.

In most ethnography reported in journal articles, however, explicit analysis strategies are not detailed. Given that ethnographic analysis is lengthy and complex, there simply is not enough space for reporting this process in the usual journal manuscript. Examination of ethnographic reports on nursing and health care shows several sources of confusion regarding data analysis. Some reports are labeled as ethnographies but are analyzed using a variety of methods, not just ethnographic ones (Delaney & Ames, 1993; Gagliari, 1991; Magilvy et al., 1987; Wing, 1990). There is no rule that says this cannot be done; in fact, the data and the purpose of the study may justify use of multiple strategies of analysis. However, it is still confusing for the neophyte researcher. In other publications, terms such as *coding, concepts, categories,* and *themes* are used without defining their specialized processes and concepts (Engebretson, 1996; Floyd, 1993; Kulig, 1995). Reports that used the strategies posed by Spradley (1979) were clearest in their steps of analysis, but even these investigators used different aspects of the Spradley methods (Connelly, Keele, Kleinbeck, & Schneider, 1993; Holland, 1993; MacDonald, 1996).

In this chapter, we first present an overview of the principles of ethnographic analysis. We then describe strategies used in the analytic process with specific examples from our research. We include a brief discussion of computerized programs and numerical methods that may prove helpful in answering specific ethnographic questions. We conclude the chapter with information about writing the report or manuscript for publication.

OVERVIEW OF ETHNOGRAPHIC ANALYSIS

Because of the nature of ethnographic data, you collect copious amounts of notes about what people do, what they say during interviews, and your personal reflections about your experiences. You may also have data from documents that you want to sift through, consolidate, and understand. Allow yourself plenty of time to perform these steps. Qualitative analysis does not "just happen." It is a process that requires rigor and investment of time and energy. Burgess (1984a) provided an example of one researcher who classified field notes into 66 specific topics, cross-referenced these topics, and then identified seven broad categories. These categories were sorted into themes on 500 single-spaced pages of notes before the researcher left the field. This is a remarkable achievement! You may or may not be able to do that. We have learned that analysis of ethnographic information is a long and thoughtful process and requires time for reflection to achieve personal understandings of complex events and the people who perform them.

The process associated with understanding ethnographic material is inductive (Becker & Geer, 1984; Burgess, 1984a), as you begin with what you learn from the data, rather than preconceived notions about your subject matter. The information that emerges from data collection guides the kinds of questions that can be answered by the project. The analysis actually begins while data are being collected, as the researcher reflexively discovers additional themes and makes decisions to follow some avenues for more intensive investigation, while ignoring less promising aspects of the project. The formal ethnographic analytic process begins with a primary identification and classification of the material that is gathered and progresses to more abstract generalizations as you discover and explain patterns of behavior and rules of the cultural group. Conducting inductive analyses require immersion in the material to gain these insights. You immerse yourself by frequently reviewing your written records of what group participants say and do and your responses while in the research environment. The systematic review of these records is the key to ethnographic data analysis.

In the next section, we present information that we found useful while analyzing our own ethnographic records. The procedures we recommend are derived from a number of sources and then consolidated into basic steps that we believe simplify, yet embrace the techniques advocated by other researchers and us. These steps are *coding* field notes and interviews, *sorting* to identify patterns, *generalizing* constructs and theories, and *memoing* to note personal reflections and insights. With the exception of memoing, we describe each step as if there were a linear process in the analysis. In reality, there is nothing linear about the analysis of ethnographic data. You move back and forth among the steps. Although memoing is described as though it occurs last, it actually does not; it happens continually as you move through the analysis. Your memoing notes are your thoughts about the data that, combined with your coding, lead to the final development of patterns and concepts. These steps are described and then illustrated with examples from our own research.

STRATEGIES OF ETHNOGRAPHIC ANALYSIS

CODING FOR DESCRIPTIVE LABELS

As we have previously stated, research material collected by the ethnographic method is in the form of written words. Observations, informal conversations, and examination of documents are converted into field notes, and taped interviews are transcribed. Ethnographic data analysis examines these words, which are first grouped into meaningful segments and then organized to compare, contrast, and identify patterns that shed light on beliefs and practices of the people in your study.

First-level coding helps you condense and reduce your many pages of data to a manageable size. Codes are descriptive labels you assign to segments or "chunks" of words, sentences, or paragraphs (Miles & Huberman, 1994), which are first examined individually and later combined to generate broader and more abstract categories. Because these descriptive codes summarize the content of the segments, they also serve a "housekeeping" role by allowing you to retrieve all information related to a specific topic.

How does coding begin? The kinds of labels used to code data depend upon the nature of your project. Codes may be assigned to answer specific research questions and may also reflect unexpected questions or concepts that emerge during the conduct of the ethnography. Generally, it is helpful to formulate basic domains that can categorize a broad range of phenomena when you are beginning the coding process (Bogdan & Biklen, 1992; Lincoln & Guba, 1985; Lofland, 1971; Miles & Huberman, 1994; Strauss, 1987; Strauss & Corbin, 1990), including

1. *Setting*: the environment or surroundings that put your site within a larger context, such as the physical space of the ICU and the people found there

2. *Activities*: behaviors or actions within the setting that occur regularly, such as bathing patients

3. *Events*: specific activities that occur infrequently, such as patient death

4. *Relationships and social structure*: patterns in the way people bond together, such as friendships, cliques, enemy relationships, and coalitions

5. *General perspectives*: group members' shared understandings of the ways things are normally done, such as care of patients after open heart surgery

6. *Specific perspectives related to the research topic*: how people understand the phenomenon of research interest, such as why patients become agitated in the ICU

7. *Strategies*: ways of accomplishing goals, such as interaction between nurses and physicians

8. *Process*: flow of events, how things change over time, or transitions, such as training of novice nurses

9. *Meanings*: what people say about the significance of their behavior, such as why nurses say they leave the ICU

10. *Repeated phrases*: comments made regularly depict patterns in thought, such as "It's a zoo in here today"

Another way to determine where to begin analysis is by examining existing documents (Morse, 1984; Magilvy et al., 1987; Roper, 1994•••). In JR's study of restraints of psychiatric patients, patient records were examined that described the restraint episode, including preceding events and behaviors of patients before, during, and after the application of restraints. Written information stated the reason and length of time that each patient remained in restraints. These data indicated that time in restraints and types of restraints used were inconsistent across patients and times of day. For example, the records revealed that one patient was placed into the most restrictive form of restraint on the evening shift but the least restrictive type on the day shift for similar behavior. This information led JR to examine and code her field notes and interview transcripts for explanations about these differences while she

TABLE 7.1   Examples of Coding Two Interviews

Question: Tell me about your feelings when you care for a patient with AD.

PATTERNS
Keep
expectations
"real"/adults

Satisfaction/
pleasure

Answer 1: I enjoy the patients. I think your *enjoyment* depends on your *expectations* of patients. If they are very high, of their recovery, you may not have satisfaction. However, if your satisfaction comes from giving comfort and not *expecting* recovery, you will get enormous *satisfaction* from working with AD patients. I understand their illness and how life for them will get no better—I think that is why they do not upset me. In fact, I get a lot of *pleasure* from working with them. I see their little idiosyncrasies that make them human and I *enjoy* getting to know them in that way. I try to see the humor in situations. I am used to having gratification from small things, so just that I think I'm making someone more comfortable is *satisfaction*. I think I know what I'm doing so that *satisfies me*. Working with these patients gives me a real sense of achievement. I don't find it particularly stressful; I rather like the work. That's why I've stayed in it for so long.

MEMOING
Look at other
interviews for
realism/
satisfaction

PATTERNS
Expect them
to act like
kids/babies

Control issue?

Frustration/
dissatisfied?

Something
should be
done

Answer 2: Just like any other patients—it's no different, they're just *like kids* almost, and we just have to take care of them *like you do kids*—do everything for them—but they don't put a whole lot of demands on you and that is good That is one good thing about them: they don't say: you're not doing this right or that wrong they never say why didn't you do this. They don't complain. They say thank you. But it makes me *tired, real tired*. If they get out of control, I just *tie them to a chair*. It takes a lot of strength to try to hold these people, to get them into chair, or change them. Sometimes you get hit. Sometimes you feel like *you haven't done enough* or done what you were supposed to do because they become agitated— you wonder if you had done this or that maybe this wouldn't have happened. I do *get frustrated*

MEMOING:
What are the
contrasts
between
interviews?

Is this
burnout?

TABLE 7.1   Continued

---

because the patients never seem to get better.
They are like *babies*. You have to go look at them
and try to see what's wrong, sometimes they can't
tell—they are crying and they can't tell you. I
feel so sad for them because *they remind me of my
grandfather*. I helped take care of him, but it was
so hard to do that. It does get to you after a while—
but it's something that *can't be helped*.

---

was still in the field. She examined her field notes for information specific to staff differences on evening and day shifts; interviews were coded for varying perceptions of staff related to specific patients and to behaviors in general. In addition, staff were asked direct questions about their attitudes toward restraints, such as when they should be used and what behaviors led to what level of restraint. It became obvious that the key to understanding restraint usage was specific patient characteristics: Patients viewed as "predictable" by the staff were perceived as needing the least restrictive devices, and patients identified as "less predictable" received the most restrictive restraints.

In Table 7.1, we present excerpts from our agitation study data to demonstrate our process of coding. We selected responses from an open-ended question that we asked nurse participants. Again, please be reminded that even though the analysis in the table looks as if it occurs in a stepwise manner, it does not. You will also note that most of our codes have to do with meaning. Nurse caregivers expressed the meaning of caring for Alzheimer's patients through their feelings.

As a first-level coding, we underlined key words that seemed to represent the feelings of these two nurse caregivers. In the interviews, we noted the repeated use of words such as *enjoyment, pleasure, satisfaction, tired, frustrated* and treating patients *like adults* or *babies or kids*. We identified in the left-hand margin the patterns that seemed to emerge from the underlined words. You may code by paragraph or section of transcribed material. Begin with broad codes that may then be broken into smaller concepts or ideas. Try to keep the number of codes to a manageable few. There is fluidity in this process. The codes are not set in concrete, and you may change your ideas about what you are seeing, hearing, and sensing over time. Document the changes in coding and reasons for the changes in your notes/memos to yourself.

These steps take time. You will be surprised at how your sleep and waking hours become occupied with understanding and interpreting the data that have been saved in your own memory banks. We have experienced revelations about data when taking showers, exercising, awakening from sleep, or even on the commute to and from work. A paper and pencil should be kept readily available for these "lightbulb" experiences.

No matter how you decide to assign descriptive labels to segments of the written material during the first-level coding process, remember that the goal is to separate the data into smaller chunks that have meaning within your specific research context. Then you are able to group or cluster the information represented by these labels to identify common phrases, patterns, and themes and also to distinguish differences between subgroups present in the cultural setting.

SORTING FOR PATTERNS

The next step in ethnographic analysis, then, is to sort or group the descriptive labels into a smaller number of sets. Each of these pattern categories incorporates several discrete codes and becomes more general and abstract as patterns explaining regularities in behaviors and beliefs emerge. Patterns become apparent as data are sorted into groupings or piles of "things [that] are alike or unlike each other" (Miles & Huberman, 1994, p. 248). You begin to develop themes that fit the data you have collected, get a more global picture of why things happen as they do, and explain recurring relationships between people in your study. You get a sense of possible connections between information you have learned, and you formulate preliminary hunches or hypotheses that are tested by asking "if-then" questions during continued participant observation.

In Table 7.1, the left-hand column represents our ideas about the patterns that emerged from the two interview questions. Note that we present only a small sample of responses; our interpretations are based on our understandings from all of the participants in our study. In the first interview, we identified the patterns of *feeling good* and *realistic patients expectations*. The pattern distinguished in the second interview reflects feelings of *frustration* and *control issues.* These patterns reflect similarities and differences between the interviews. Questions we asked ourselves during this process were: (a) Are the similarities enough alike to represent a true pattern? (b) Do the differences reflect extraordinary responses ("outliers"), or are there shared characteristics in the differences? We also asked ourselves about the patterns' relationships to already established concepts, such as burnout and stress. We wondered if the patterns represented a stage in the process leading to burnout or stress. We further compared these patterns to descriptions in the literature related to burnout and stress.

OUTLIERS

At any step in your analysis, you may identify cases, situations, events, or settings that do not "fit" with the rest of your findings. Do not discard these outliers, but use them to test the rest of your data. They may strengthen your analysis and offer information that will lead to a better understanding and explanation of your findings (Miles & Huberman, 1994, p. 269). In our agitation study, we identified two cases that seemed to not fit the patterns that we discovered from the interviews and that were not congruent with the field notes from our observations. These cases were two staff members who viewed patients very differently from other staff. They were more negative toward patients and, without caution, admitted to the use of restraints as the only way of managing patients. In addition, they were generally pessimistic about the hospital and the ward, yet they felt confident that their actions were correct and benefited the patients. This was a strange mix of confidence and negativism. We kept these two cases in mind as we developed the different steps in analysis. When we were unsure about others in our study, we used these two cases for comparison and contrast. Because of their outlier features, they were the exception that provided support for our analysis and understanding of the total patterns of responses.

Thus far, we have labeled discrete segments of the data with descriptive codes and explored relationships between categories by identifying patterns of regularities. The next step continues the search for even more abstractions that explain and link understandings to constructs or theories that may emerge from the data.

TABLE 7.2 Data Matrix for Study on Agitation in Alzheimer's Disease: Characteristics of Nurse Caregivers

Subject No.	Gender	Age (Years)	Position	Helpless/ Hopeless	Confident	Satisfied	Frustrated
1	F	42	RN	Yes	No	Not sure	Yes
2	F	59	NA	Yes	No	Yes	Yes
3	M	30	NA	No	Yes	No	Yes
4	M	36	RN	No	Yes	Yes	No
5	M	60	LVN	Yes	No	No	Yes
6	F	52	RN	Not sure	Yes	Yes	Not sure

GENERALIZING: CONSTRUCTS AND THEORIES

A significant aim of ethnographic analysis is to discover an ever-expanding and ever more abstract network of interrelated concepts to explain the events and activities that you are told about or that you witness through ethnographic methods. You want to connect these findings to theories that make sense of the rich and complex data you collect. To generalize findings about the cultural world of study, find linkages between the emic meanings and worldview of study participants and your etic interpretations of those meanings, and then construct theoretical understandings that take both of these perspectives into account. It is helpful to develop a data matrix to display the relationships between descriptive codes, patterns, and emerging theory. Refer to Table 7.2 for an example of a data matrix from our agitation study. We sorted the participants in the study by a number of variables: gender, age, position, and various feelings such as helplessness, confidence, satisfaction, and frustration. A "yes" in a column indicates that that participant shares the feeling. A "no" means that we did not find that feeling stated in the interview. A question mark indicates that we were not sure if the feeling was present or not. When all responses from participants are entered into a data matrix, it is often easier to discern specific patterns and their relationships.

In our agitation study, we reflected on the patterns from the coding process. We identified nurses who saw themselves as personally involved in the care of Alzheimer's disease (AD) patients and treated them like relatives. We also found nurses who were dissatisfied with the care they gave and felt hopeless and helpless while working with agitated patients. Other nurses saw themselves as more objective and able to view the patient in a realistic perspective, not expecting more of the patient than what was determined by the illness; these nurses seemed to be satisfied with the care they gave and confident in their caregiving style. We examined several possible concepts that might explain the perceptions of these nurses in dealing with agitation in AD patients. One of these concepts was "burnout." Could nurses be experiencing burnout as they managed the care of the AD patients' agitation day after day? Our nurse caregivers presented some of the characteristics of staff who are burned out. We reviewed the literature on burnout, but we were not convinced that burnout truly represented what the nurses were telling us. The literature on family caregivers indicates that stress, burden, and depression are commonly found among family caregivers of Alzheimer's patients. We reviewed this literature and in fact recoded and sorted our interview data to look for evidence of these emotional responses. This exercise did not help us in understanding the perceptions of the nurse caregivers. The work in defining a concept was finally achieved by a marathon session where we reflected on the words of the nurse caregivers and performed a final organization of the patterns into two separate distinctions. It was then that a concept of "distancing," became very apparent and applicable to all cases (except for the two outliers discussed earlier).

MEMOING: REFLECTIVE REMARKS

Memos are ideas or insights you have about the data. They are a form of coding that is done as you collect data and review interviews, observations, and relevant documents. They often pull together notations that have commonalties and allow you to make connections between pieces of information. They may be questions you ask yourself or "little conceptual epiphanies" (Miles & Huberman, 1994, p. 74) that later lead to theoretical understandings. Memos are written so that you can readily recognize that they are reflections needing further testing and not objective material that was observed or heard. We prefer to italicize all of our memos to ourselves. These reflections occur during all stages of data collection and analysis and provide the basis for deep and meaningful understandings of your data. The right-hand column of Table 7.1 represents memos to ourselves as we analyzed the data. Later, these thoughts were used to question our understanding of the data and provide direction for further exploration of our study and supporting literature.

The restraint study conducted by Roper (Roper & Anderson, 1991) provided an example of memoing. The term *control* was frequently used by both patients and staff of the psychiatric unit. JR became aware of this as she reviewed interview data and the patient record documentation. She had not seen this term in the literature on restraints, nor had she heard staff use the word in any other context. She made a note of the word *control* when it appeared, with the questions of "What does this mean in terms of restraint usage?" and "Do all staff and patients mean the same thing when they talk about control?" She also wanted to know more about the issue of control for staff. "Do staff always have to be in control? What does that mean for restraint usage? What do patients think of control?" These questions that she had memoed from interviews and observations then provided another focus for her inquiries and observations. Control was important for both staff and patients. Staff needed to feel in control of the environment. They did not want patient behavior to get to the point where staff could no longer effectively manage the ward safely and therapeutically. Patients respected staff for their ability to control the ward and were concerned if staff let it get out of control. These deep and complex meanings of the word *control* were identified and understood through this reflective process.

GENERAL COMMENTS

In sum, analysis of ethnographic material is both process and procedure. It is a process of breaking up or segmenting your raw data into small bits and pieces and then reassembling them into patterns or wholes (Jorgensen, 1989). You begin the process by coding your field notes, interviews, and document data. You seek comparisons and contrasts. You ask various questions as you sort the information to validate your labels and patterns. Summarizing and displaying your findings in a data matrix makes it easier to formulate constructs and theories as conclusions are drawn. You develop methods to summarize or display your analysis. Interpretations are then made that convert emic information to etic understanding. This often takes the form of description in your report.

We repeat that the analysis does not happen in an orderly fashion. It is not linear but moves back and forth among the activities of coding, memoing, sorting for patterns, and generalizing. You may feel that you need to get answers from your data right away, but it is best to not get locked into patterns too quickly, as you may miss additional understandings from paths not traveled.

Keep a paper trail of your analysis. You will need to be able to explain to others how you formulated your final concepts. Though ethnographic studies are generally not replicated, you should still be able to articulate your analytic steps, when you did them, and how you did them. You and others will want to be assured that your ethnography is firmly grounded in sound analytic strategies that represent good science.

Finally, keep copies of your raw data and steps in analysis in safe places. Your whole study will be lost without that information. If you use a computer program for data analysis, be sure to keep back up copies on diskettes. If you rely on the typewritten/handwritten methods, also make copies of the data and analysis process. Store them in different places, just in case something happens to one copy. Unfortunately, with the paper method, you fell many trees, but eventually the copies can be recycled.

COMPUTER TECHNOLOGIES

TEXT ANALYSIS USING COMPUTERS

Ethnographic research relies on written text compiled from field notes of observations and transcribed interviews from research participants. These written documents can be analyzed by "hand," but specialized computer software programs may more easily manage the volume of information. Approximately two dozen computer programs are available to help you code, retrieve, and analyze your data (Miles & Huberman, 1994). Weitzman and Miles (1994) have discussed specific features of the most popular programs. Bernard and Ryan (1998) also

---

TABLE 7.3   Selected Software Programs

---

1. Atlas/ti
2. QSR NUD*IST
3. The Ethnograph
4. Code-A-Text

Information for these four programs is available through:
    Scolari, Sage Publications, Inc.
    2455 Teller Road
    Thousand Oaks, CA 91320
    (805) 499-1325
    e-mail: scolari@sagepub.com
    http://www.scolari.com

5. Kwalitan
    Qualitative Research Management
    73-425 Hilltop Road
    Desert Hot Springs, CA 92241-7821
    (619) 329-7026
    e-mail: Hallock_Hoffman@mcimail.com

---

have described useful strategies of computer-assisted text analysis and have provided concrete examples from published studies. Table 7.3 provides a list of selected programs with their mail and e-mail addresses. They are reviewed in detail over the Internet, and some allow you to download demonstration programs. In addition to reviewing these descriptions, talk to colleagues and mentors for their suggestions.

Though we are still novices in computerized text analysis, we appreciate the potential of these powerful data management tools. On the most basic level, the majority of these programs allow the researcher to label segments of text with codes and later to retrieve passages of texts surrounding these codes. For example, in the study pertaining to the impact of agitated patient behaviors on ICU nurses, JS noted that these nurses employ the term *control* in various ways. Examining the sentences before and after *control* helped her identify distinct patterns in the beliefs and practices of the ICU nurses. Many programs also have the ability to tabulate the number of times a particular word is used in a body of text. This feature may help distinguish differences between members of a cultural group, such as women and men, patients and doctors, or senior and junior nurses. From these patterns in coded labels, concepts are developed.

Computerized analysis programs are further used to identify relationships among emerging concepts. One of the questions that has evolved from the ongoing ICU study is the relationship between nurse agitation and patient agitation: Do nurses report more patient agitation when they feel "out of control" for non-patient-related reasons (i.e., administrative demands or personal problems)? Programs with the ability to perform *semantic network analysis* or *cognitive mapping* may help JS determine which concepts precede other concepts in the minds and actions of study participants.

It is important to understand that these software programs depend upon *your* interpretation of the research data: You supply the codes that give meaning to the text and provide the intuition for linking patterns into concepts and relationships. Computers help organize this information and are efficient in performing automatic tasks. Be sure to budget time (and patience) in your schedule to learn how to run the program you select. And it is extremely helpful to network with other researchers using the same program(s) to share tips and horrors!

QUANTIFYING ETHNOGRAPHIC DATA

Computers and their appropriate software applications are essential when you use numerical or quantitative methods to enhance understanding of your data. Unlike qualitative analyses, which involve ongoing and continual examination, quantitative analyses are generally conducted at the conclusion of the project. We highly recommend that you obtain a general understanding of statistical methods and consultation with a statistician *before* data collection begins to ensure that data can be analyzed sensibly after fieldwork is ended. Although it is beyond the scope of this book to detail specific quantitative analysis strategies, we provide examples of the kinds of ethnographic questions that may be answered with numerical procedures, as well as names of corresponding statistical tests. A recent discussion by Handwerker and Borgatti (1998) helped us organize our comments for this section.

Ethnographers observe and survey their domain of study. As we advocate in Chapter 6, be specific when collecting information about the setting, people, and variables of interest. Count when possible: the number of men and women, ages of the participants, people in the waiting room, houses in the community, or beds in the hospital ward. You can then supply a general picture and identify patterns in the way people think and behave using *descriptive statistics*. It is helpful to determine the *mode* for variables, or what the majority of participants do/are, and also the *mean* of variables of interest for the population, such as the average age at first pregnancy, average number of years living in the country, or average number of minutes that nurse managers spend with patients. You can also identify the relative placement of an event or process by computing the *median*, or middle point along a distribution, and learn if what you observe is typical in the community. For example, if you want to know the general socioeconomic status of a group of family caregivers of patients with Alzheimer's disease, arrange their annual incomes from lowest to highest, and then mark the middle or median value; this statistic is useful when there are extreme scores in a set, such as one millionaire among a group of people eligible for financial assistance. In addition to identifying these averages, or what typically happens, you can evaluate variations in behavioral and cognitive patterns. You can identify how common something is, such as beliefs about the cause of an illness, by counting the number of individuals who endorse specific views; this is called a *frequency*. The point of view with the highest count is the *modal frequency*. This number is usually given as a *percentage* (modal frequency divided by total number · 100) or as a *ratio* (the number of people who express one belief system divided by the number of people with any other belief system). The variation in patterns within a population is statistically measured by the *standard deviation*. A large variation implies that many circumstances influence how people think and behave, whereas little variation suggests meaningful controls on divergent views and behavior (Handwerker & Borgatti, 1998). If there are many ways of thinking, such that, for example, only 20% of the people express the most common or modal view, we can presume a high degree of cultural diversity. Conversely, if 80% of study participants endorse the modal belief, we may conclude that a cultural consensus exists for the concept (Handwerker & Borgatti, 1998).

Consensus analysis (Romney, Weller, & Batchelder, 1986; Weller, 1987) is a method used by researchers to answer an important ethnographic question: Who agrees with whom about what and to what degree? (Handwerker & Borgatti, 1998, p. 569). Other strategies that help you decide which events and processes "go together" from those that do not are *factor analysis, cluster analysis,* and *multidimensional scaling.* These statistical tools convert the immense number of relationships detailed in your field notes into graphic maps that can be more readily interpreted. The ANTHROPAC software program is specifically designed to model patterns of agreement and relationships within a cultural domain (Borgatti, 1992). JS will use these methods to identify shared nursing beliefs about agitation and to describe the complex relationship between beliefs and actions in the ICU.

Depending upon the type of data collected, you might want to generalize findings from your study to a larger population. This *inferential data analysis* is the hallmark of quantitative statistics and is contingent upon measuring characteristics from a random or unbiased sample of independent cases or individuals. Examples of these classical statistical tests are chi-squares and *t* tests. Information from existing documents may include variables appropriate for inferential statistics. Shapira (1997) used inferential statistics to analyze differences in care received by psychiatric and nonpsychiatric patients in an emergency department. Before the study, there was general staff consensus that psychiatric patients waited longer than medical patients. Tabulating the number of minutes and hours that a random sample of patients spent in the emergency department clearly demonstrated that psychiatric patients as a group stayed significantly shorter periods of time than nonpsychiatric patients. Ethnographic observations and staff interviews provided explanations for this discrepancy.

In conclusion, computers and accompanying software programs are increasingly used to analyze both textual and numerical ethnographic data. These powerful tools help you to more easily identify patterns and variances among people and events captured in your field notes. Allow time to experiment with these programs to determine which fit best with your research questions before starting data collection. Obtain consultation from knowledgeable colleagues and mentors. And remember that you are the key to data analysis: You determine the initial and ongoing questions, interpret what you learn, and assign meaning to the rich complexities of subjective and objective experiences inherent in ethnographic research.

WRITING THE PAPER

If you are reading this book, you are probably readying yourself to conduct your ethnographic study. You will write not only to complete your research proposal but to share your research with others. According to Wolcott (1990), there are writers and there are readers, and rarely is one person equally good at both activities. But the reality is that readers, especially those, who do research, must write (Morse & Field, 1995). As a student, that became obvious very early in your academic career. Often academic experiences convince students that they are not writers, and once out of school, they swear not to write another paper.

Writing is hard for most people (Fetterman, 1989). Though reading is a passive activity that you can plug into wherever you are, writing requires goal-directed behavior. There is a professional obligation that if you conduct research, you must let people know about it. You even have to let them know about your failures or studies that do not work out exactly as expected. The purpose of this section, then, is to provide you with some information about writing in general and then with more specifics about writing for publication.

WRITING IN GENERAL

Do not put off your writing (Wolcott, 1990). It is quite easy to say, "I know what I am going to write—it is in my head." We are all probably guilty of this statement from time to time. There is something intimidating about putting your thoughts to paper. First of all, some order, organization, and discipline is required. JR has tried to write in 20- or 30-minute segments of time; this generally works only for short reports and will not work for lengthy research papers. However, these short periods of time can be used to draw up an outline that you can use later when you have more time.

Find protected time and a comfortable place to write. These days, most often, it is in front of a computer, but there is nothing wrong with the yellow legal-size tablet and a pencil or pen. JR does both. If she is having trouble with a paragraph or a section, she goes back to the tried and true—paper and pencil. The computer just doesn't seem as amenable. We all joke about eating around the computer. Wolcott (1990) talked about triscuits and cheese; our colleagues try to find less calorie-loaded goodies to munch on. JR just makes sure there is cold water or hot tea close by.

In your protected time, just write. It is best *not* to edit while you are writing. You can edit later. Many people get stuck in the writing phase of their research because they try to make the first version the only version. This does not work! Use your outline, if that works for you as you write, but do not try to make every sentence perfect and every paragraph meaningful. You can do that later.

Stay focused on the reason for writing the paper. Wolcott (1990) recommended writing the purpose on a paper and always having that in view when you are writing. It is easy to go off on tangents without realizing that you have moved from your original purpose.

Identify friends or colleagues who will read what you have written after you have a version of the paper that satisfies you. Sometimes you have friends who are very forgiving and will read very early versions of a paper and give you excellent feedback. We have found, however, that it is best to ask colleagues to review a paper closer to completion than an early rough draft. Remember, also, that a paper goes through many drafts. Save these drafts until the final version is completed. The personal computer is extremely valuable in redrafting versions, as well as in saving the prior versions of a paper.

WRITING YOUR RESEARCH PAPER

The ultimate goal of putting your research into writing is to get it published. You may also, however, have to write a report as part of your funding contract; the agency where you conducted the research may want a report; and subjects may request a copy of your report. What we say in this section, however, is directed at writing for publication. Certainly, some of the same principles apply for the other purposes as well.

Some anthropologists have written their ethnographies while in the field (Sanjek, 1990). The material is fresh, and the participants in the study are available for feedback. Generally, however, ethnographic writing is done away from the field. Experienced researchers recommend that you start your writing *before* you conduct your study. In fact, one investigator who does primarily quantitative research writes at least one complete paper before the study is started. It may have to be modified pending results, but that is far easier than starting from scratch. For ethnographic researchers, such a procedure may not be possible or advisable. What can be done early is the section that describes the background of the study and the projected methodology. The literature review can be started and continually updated as the study is in process. The results section must wait for the completion of your study.

You will want to write ethnographic research so that the reader can share in your experiences. Thus, quotations are frequently used to give the reader firsthand information. You may take some license with your transcriptions to make them flow with the rest of the narrative. Make sure you present the information so that research participants cannot be identified. You may want to present some of your findings in tables. Diagrams and other illustrative methods enhance your document (Morse & Field, 1995).

Write in the active voice. Take out verbs that are passive. Keep your paper alive for the reader. Write in the first person unless otherwise instructed by the respective journal. This issue has not been settled in the research arena, so some journals still require the third person for all writing.

Look for the possible publishing source appropriate for your paper. Read those journals and review their criteria for publication submissions. Who reads the journal? Is it a clinical or research journal? Your paper should be written for a specific audience. You can even query the journal editor to ascertain their interest in your paper. Follow the guidelines for the journal you have selected for submission of your manuscript. Submit to only one journal at a time. Be sure to follow the rules religiously. Journals will reject papers, without reviewing them, for not following guidelines.

Try to publish in a peer-reviewed journal—one that has a review panel beyond the editorial board that reviews and critiques papers. Most research-focused journals are peer reviewed.

If your study was conducted with other researchers, decide on authorship issues early in the study development. Misunderstandings about authorship have resulted in angry feelings and missed opportunities. The principal investigator on the study does not have to be first author on all papers. Decide on your criteria for determining authorship. Some possible criteria: The first author is one who does the most work on the paper or came up with the idea for the study, or the first author is the one who needs a paper for promotion/vitae.

Do not be surprised if you get rejected on the first try. It is common for papers to be returned to the author with recommendations for revisions. Some journals indicate whether they would reconsider the paper with the appropriate revisions. Sometimes the journal staff value the paper and offer assistance in editing from their editorial staff. All of this depends on the specific publication. If you have not heard from the journal in 3 months after submission of your manuscript, contact them and get some feedback regarding the status of the paper. Journal companies have been known to lose manuscripts. This is another reason to save copies on a diskette and to make hard copies as well.

Many journals will want the revised manuscript on a diskette for publication. That diskette will not be returned to you. Be sure to read the guidelines for specifications of font size, margins, spacing, and citations. If a diskette copy is required and a specific word-processing program is specified, follow those instructions.

Many nurses hire typists or even editors to assist them with their papers. We really like to do our own initial typing of the paper because we think while writing and often gain new insights from that process. If you do your own typing, you can give it to a typist or editor when you have finished to put the final touches on the manuscript. Others cannot type and find they have to do their revisions in other ways. Whatever system you use, make it work for you.

SUMMARY

This chapter has dealt with the complex process of analyzing ethnographic data. Guidelines for organizing and understanding the information collected through the fieldwork experience were presented. We discussed the application of computer technologies and relevant software programs for data management, textual analysis, and numerical reasoning. Important points to remember are:

- Ethnographic analysis involves the processes of coding, identifying patterns, generalizing, making reflective memos, and formulating concepts. These processes are not linear. They do not happen in a specific order.

- Computers can be used in ethnographic analysis. The success of this process depends upon your identification of meaningful codes, patterns, and meanings from interviews and field notes.

- Ethnographic data can be viewed and analyzed quantitatively. Careful characterization of specific events, situations, and people contributes to the richness of your findings.

- Publishing your study and the results is part of the ethnographic research process. It is your professional obligation.

8

ETHICAL RESPONSIBILITIES

This above all: to thine own self be true,
And it must follow as the night the day,
Thou canst not then be false to any man.
Shakespeare, *Hamlet,* (Act I, Scene 3,
cited in Bartlett 1968, p. 259a)

Conducting ethnography is a personal experience as the investigator "lives" alongside the participants of the study and moves from being a complete stranger to being a quasi-member of the group. Because you listen to their stories, accept explanations of how members see the world, and share physical and emotional experiences together, a relationship develops between investigator and informants that is unlike that found in other research designs. This personal involvement during data collections extends to the formal analysis phase of the project, in which interpretations are scrutinized and linked together in a coherent whole.

Investigators have significant ethical responsibilities during the conduct of *any* project to both study participants and consumers of final reports. Two features of ethnographic research create particular ethical concern: This paradigm is based upon personal interaction between ethnographers and group members, and investigators themselves are the primary data collection instruments (Brink, 1993, p. 238; Cassell, 1992, p. 31; Morse & Field, 1995, p. 141). Researchers using this methodology are constantly aware of the potential for ethical dilemmas, and they adopt specific strategies to address these issues. First, they deliberately evaluate their own effects on the research process by consciously identifying biases brought to the field and also emotional responses resulting from their experiences. Next, they come up with an explicit description of their role during data collection. Finally, they establish mechanisms that guarantee honest and trustworthy research relationships. For the purpose of discussion, these approaches are presented separately, but in reality they are intertwined and can occur during any stage of the research process.

IDENTIFICATION OF BIASES

Ethnographers recognize that their work is always comparative, for "the student of culture is himself 'cultured' " (Manheim, 1936, cited in Werner & Schoepfle, 1987, p. 172). Investigators bring to the field their own identities and life experiences (Kleinman & Copp, 1993, p. 10). These expectations influence what is "seen" and carry the risk that investigators will merely project *their* perceptions onto informants' statements and actions without acquiring a valid account of salient beliefs and systems of meaning of the group members. Steps can be taken to counteract these possibilities before and during data collection.

In preparation for your research experience, learn to be receptive to differences. Read extensively about other cultures, and acquire an appreciation for the wide variation in the way individuals think and behave. Search out opportunities to personally experience new surroundings and activities. Consider spending time with immigrant groups or people of a different economic status from your own. By noticing what seems strange in these encounters, you identify taken-for-granted aspects of your personal perspective.

Obtain an awareness of potential "blind spots" (Werner & Schoepfle, 1987, p. 170) or personal baggage that must be honestly acknowledged. Kleinman and Copp (1993) suggested:

Ask yourself about the needs you expect this setting to fulfill: Do I have an axe to grind? Do I have a mission? Am I looking for a cause or a community? Do I expect this study to help me resolve personal problems? Am I hoping to create a different self? What political assumptions do I have? What kinds of settings or activities or subgroups might I avoid or discount because of who or what I am? (p. 58)

It is helpful to write the answers to these questions in your personal journal before entering the setting. You can then review them when discrepancies between your expectations and observations occur and use them to determine the degree that personal bias may be influencing your interpretations.

Recognize that strong feelings, both positive and negative, are common while doing ethnography. Acknowledge these feelings, and use them to explain what you learn. Jean Briggs (1970), who lived with a group of Utku Eskimos for 1 year, clearly and poignantly described her own feelings in particular situations. For example, as an adopted "daughter" of one family, she was expected to follow the orders of the "father," a situation that resulted in much tension for her. Through intensive analysis of her notes after leaving the field, she realized that much of the stress she had felt in the situation had been caused by reminders of the relationship with her own family and her need for personal independence.

This awareness of the dynamic interaction between the investigator and the research environment is called reflexivity (Marcus & Fischer, 1986). Reflexivity includes careful consideration of the reciprocal exchange between the ethnographer and study participants. The process requires deliberate self-awareness and direction of conscious attention to reasons behind one's particular responses to people and events. In addition, it requires taking into account the ongoing influence of the investigator's personal characteristics, cultural belief systems, and physical presence during data collection and interpretation of findings from the study.

Nurse researchers have the added task of examining values and beliefs that are derived from their socialization and experiences as nurses (Lamb & Huttlinger, 1989). This is most significant when working within one's own culture or peer group. Lipson (1984) explored the subjective experience of cesarean birth with women who attended two mutual support groups. In this study, she combined the roles of anthropologist-researcher, nurse-clinician, and peer after having cesarean births herself. She actively participated in group discussions and conducted private in-depth interviews with other members. Lipson was acutely aware of potential biases in the study and carefully documented the interaction between her feelings and the research process in a personal diary. Though she noted minor difficulties associated with separating the researcher and participant roles and some problems in recognizing patterns among familiar behaviors, she concluded that the use of these perspectives enriched the quality of the data she collected.

The goal of ethnography is to determine the perspective of *all* participants in the research setting, including the investigator. Identifying personal, cultural, and professional belief systems before entering the field site and maintaining distinct records of emotional responses to persons and events during data collection help manage potential sources of biases influencing the research process.

INSIDER/OUTSIDER ROLE

The role of the investigator doing ethnography is complex for both researcher and group members. Ideally, a strategy is found that allows the investigator to participate fully in activities as an *insider* while consciously and objectively describing and analyzing the events as an *outsider*. According to Hammersley and Atkinson (1983), "There must always remain some part held back, some social and intellectual 'distance.' For it is in the 'space' created by this distance that the analytic work of the ethnographer gets done" (p. 102). This requisite distancing keeps the ethnographer always marginal to group members (Shaffir & Stebbins, 1991, p. 21). The degree of marginality, however, must be carefully considered, as the perception of the researcher by group members affects what they share about themselves and their culture. The quality of the information and the depth of analysis depend on the researcher's ability to establish trust and gain rapport.

It is difficult to be an outsider, particularly when moving to an unfamiliar environment. Researchers may experience feelings of "culture shock" similar to those experienced by immigrants of a new country or patients admitted to a hospital for "foreign" medical procedures. Brink and Saunders (1976) related the period of adjustment to multiple

changes to various categories of stressors, including the effects of isola-
tion, communication difficulty, and differences in customs, attitudes,
and beliefs. It is not uncommon for researchers to feel lonely, particularly at the beginning of a project. Capture these feelings in the personal
diary, and analyze how emotional responses could shape the interpretations made during this interval. Another helpful strategy is to collect
concrete observations that are less dependent upon emotional influences during this initial period of the project, such as a general survey
and mapping of the physical layout of the setting.

Group members you hope to study also have beliefs about your role in
their world. Ethnographers are viewed as intruders (Werner & Schoepfle, 1987, p. 257), strangers, and friends (Powdermaker, 1966). First, try
to discover their expectations of you, and clarify any discrepancies that
exist. For example, when JS first described her proposed study of agitation in the intensive care unit (ICU) to nursing staff, one nurse said,
"Good. Then you'll be able to tell the doctors we need standing orders
of which meds to give." She was grateful for that comment because it
gave her an opportunity to clarify how she perceived her role as researcher. Make sure group members understand what you will do during the research project (i.e., ask questions, observe activities, and read
documents), what kind of information you want to collect, how you will
use what has been learned, and what help you need from them (McCall
& Simmons, 1969, p. 43).

In addition to explaining the specific tasks associated with the research role, the investigator must manage personal relationships that develop with study participants. Recognize when you are considered a
friend rather than a researcher. Though it may afford a sense of belong-
ing to be treated like a confidant, it has both methodological and ethical
implications. Seed (1995) described her challenges in negotiating a comfortable role with nursing students during a 3-year ethnographic analysis of their experiences. She characterized an evolving relationship with
these student-subjects that included establishing trust, proving the ability to maintain confidentiality, and rehearsing clinical assignments.
Though Seed participated in direct patient care activities with the
student-subjects and felt accepted by them as a person, she was careful to
continually establish her primary presence as a researcher.

Ethnographers learn to balance this insider/outsider role by establishing bounded, reciprocal relationships with group members (Byerly,

1969). Lipson (1989) worked with Afghan refugees in California and helped them during appointments with the Department of Motor Vehicles and by filling out immigration forms. Kauffman (1994) participated in the lives of members of a senior center in a urban ghetto. She joined them for activities at the center and was invited to family gatherings. In return, she introduced her visiting relatives to the study participants and drove them to meetings she thought they would enjoy. The mutual relationships described by Lipson and Kauffman provided depth to their understandings as researchers while benefiting study participants. Neither investigator described conflicts in maintaining the role of researcher.

Maintaining boundaries between the insider and outsider roles becomes even more significant when working within one's own culture, where there are no clear behavioral or social signs that differentiate the researcher from study participants. The investigator has an ethical responsibility to remind group members that they are participating in a research project, and their consent is continually negotiated (Germain, 1993). Group members should have the right to decide when to share personal information. The need to safeguard the privacy of individuals is respected in the acceptable practice of public observation; though covert research is not appropriate, observing and participating in communal activities once the research role is explained are hallmarks of ethnography. The key is to respect the dignity and rights of all who come in contact with you.

In addition to balancing role responsibilities and trusting relationships with subjects, nurses must also consider their professional integrity (Seed, 1995). Though nurse-researchers may consider themselves primarily researchers, their subjects may perceive them differently. Because of their neutral positions and nonjudgmental attitudes, researchers often serve as sounding boards for nurses who become subjects of studies (Byerly, 1969, p. 232). Confusion and disappointment occur when nurse-researchers do not address administrative problems that have been brought to their attention. For example, during our work with nurses who cared for Alzheimer's disease patients, many expressed their frustration with perceived insufficient staffing patterns. Several months after completion of the study, one nurse approached JS and asked if more nurses were going to be added to the unit. When JS answered that she didn't know, the nurse responded angrily, "But I told you we needed more nurses!" We felt responsible for the misunderstanding, even though it had been explained that results from our study would not be directly shared with nursing managers; clearly, our roles as researchers were not apparent to this nurse. In other instances, nurse-researchers are granted expert status and asked to provide consultation and advice (Jackson, 1975). Field (1989) noted that although being acknowledged as a nurse is advantageous in gaining entry to the setting, it is crucial for informants to understand that the investigator is acting as a researcher and not a nurse.

Patients also become perplexed about these role differences. Anticipate these potential issues, and develop a plan to manage them. In JR's restraint and seclusion study, patients approached her and asked what she was doing on their ward. The study was explained, and patients either walked away or volunteered to tell her about restraints. Staff, on the other hand, never queried her *directly* about her role, so she initiated a discussion of her project during scheduled team meetings. In JS's ICU study, data are collected from a sample of patients before their surgeries. Patients are interviewed after the anticipated procedures have been explained and after surgical consent has been obtained by their physicians. If patients ask any questions about their surgeries, the physician and head nurse of the unit will be informed of the patients' concerns; thus, a conscious attempt is made to keep clear boundaries between the researcher role and nursing responsibilities.

A particular challenge for nurse-researchers occurs when there is a perceived need to advocate on a subject's behalf. Our greatest challenges conducting research within our nursing culture occurred when we felt a need to directly intervene with patient care. JS notified an attending physician when a resident physician obtained informed consent for an invasive procedure from a legally incompetent patient. JR observed that a patient was kept in restraints for unclear reasons and used her role as a "questioning researcher" to bring it to the attention of the head nurse. When compelled to intervene, document the situation and responses carefully in field notes, and see if a particular pattern emerges from these uncommon cases (J. Saunders, personal communication, 1994).

Lipson (1989) identified the less subtle example of responding "therapeutically" when subjects manifest distress. During our interviews with spouse caregivers of patients with Alzheimer's disease, we discovered that every spouse cried at some point during the research meeting. When this occurred, we asked if they wished to continue (all subjects agreed to finish the discussion). After the interview, we turned off the tape recorder, put down our pencils, and addressed specific concerns of the subjects. This strategy allowed us to move between our roles of researchers and clinicians. There are no rules about when to intervene or how to manage the variety of available roles; each nurse-researcher decides what is appropriate within the specific research context.

ISSUES OF INFORMED CONSENT

An individual who agrees to participate in a research project enters into a specific relationship with the investigator. The responsibility of the investigator is to clearly inform subjects of potential positive and negative consequences associated with the particular study (Lipson, 1994). General benefits of an ethnographic endeavor include an increased understanding of the individuals and groups under study, and contribution to the advancement of human knowledge (Cassell, 1980). The possibility for harmful effects from ethnographic studies are relatively minimal, involving primarily violations of privacy or confidentiality (Cassell, 1980). After the project is explained, the individual can make a knowledgeable decision about participation.

The process of obtaining informed consent from research subjects originated with the Nuremberg war trials (Burgess, 1984b, p. 200) and was designed to prevent unlawful and immoral experimentation. Currently, protection of human subjects is carefully regulated by institutional review boards in academic and medical settings and focuses on the rights of potential subjects, including an explanation of the purpose, risks, and benefits of the study; the ability to refuse participation at any time; and the protection of anonymity and confidentiality. Ethnographic studies may not require the completion of *written* consent forms, depending upon the particular methods used in the study design and the setting where the research occurs: For example, an anthropology colleague of JS works with a group of people in Peru who have no written language. Also, when a researcher is conducting participant observation of activities that occur normally in a setting and specific individuals cannot be identified from the data, formal consent is not required. If, however, interactions are videotaped or interviews are audiotaped, a written guarantee of how the information will be protected is mandatory. Regardless of whether permission from potential subjects is obtained with written contracts or verbal agreements, the investigator must provide a clear description of the research. Though the exact wording of consent forms varies among institutional settings, information is usually provided that describes the purpose of the study; how long the study will last; what the subject will be asked to do; procedures that may result in discomfort or inconvenience; expected risks; expected benefits, including financial compensation; and how the results from the project will be used.

The consent procedure poses unique dilemmas for those conducting ethnographies. Investigators may have difficulty formulating consent forms that address all aspects of the proposed research; ethnographies evolve over time, and all questions or areas to be explored may not be known before data collection is underway (Lipson, 1994). Munhall (1988) presented a concept of "process consenting" that reflects the ongoing and dynamic nature of ethnographic research. Consent is "renegotiated as unexpected events or consequences" of the project occur (p. 151).

The consent process concentrates on the rights of *individual* subjects. In ethnographies, however, the unit of analysis may be the family or small group. Lipson (1994, p. 342) raised fitting concerns about protecting the privacy of the individual during family interviews: Will information be shared by others that the individual prefers not to have told?

The method of obtaining formal, written consent may conflict with cultural practices of group members. During their work with Middle Eastern refugees, Lipson and Meleis (1989) discovered that prospective subjects were uncomfortable when the consent form was read or given to them; they felt rude when appearing distrustful of the investigators' project. The researchers avoided this problem by stating that the university insisted the document be read.

Nurses have further ethical considerations when conducting participant observation studies. We often work with vulnerable or stigmatized populations (Saunders & Valente, 1992) such as persons with AIDS, pregnant adolescents, cancer survivors, the elderly, and those with chronic mental conditions. Lee and Renzetti (1993) identified areas of investigation that may be threatening to those being studied. Clearly, care must be taken when research intrudes into private aspects of peoples' lives or involves deeply personal experiences, including financial or sexual matters or issues surrounding bereavement. Sensitive research material also results when a study is concerned with deviance or social control and the possibility that participants could be identified, stigmatized, or incriminated exists. Agar (1973) and Adler and Adler (1993) worked with people involved in illicit drug activities and were particularly careful in safeguarding the confidences shared with them. Finally, investigators struggle when confronted with information that is sacred to those being studied, such as the relationship between healing practices and religious beliefs.

The investigator confronted with sensitive topics faces a dilemma when deciding whether to present findings in academic journals or public conferences. Brink (1993) questioned if she had the right to publish what she had learned in Africa about secret women's societies; the issue remains unresolved in her mind. The informed consent process should specify what the researcher intends to do with the results of the study. It is argued, however, that subjects may not realize the full emotional impact that hearing or reading about themselves will have on them. Scheper-Hughes (1979) conducted an ethnography of a town in Ireland and published her results in an award-winning book. She returned to the town several years later and was confronted with anger and dismay from the local people. They questioned whether she had the right to discuss their lives, even though her reports were accurate (Burgess, 1984b, pp. 204-205). Though Scheper-Hughes had been careful to discuss only shared community knowledge in her book, she was told by an informant, "There is quite a difference between whispering something beside a fire or across a counter and seeing it printed for the world to see. It becomes *public* shame (Scheper-Hughes, 1981, emphasis in original, cited in Burgess, 1984b, p. 204).

Some investigators involve their subjects in the decision of what to publish about them. Judith Saunders used an informant's personal biography to understand the impact of HIV disease on his life. He actively reviewed and corrected what she wrote about him and successfully negotiated for first authorship of the article (Armendariz, Saunders, Poston, & Valente, 1997; J. Saunders, personal communication, 1996). When study participants wish to remain anonymous, extreme caution is taken to avoid publishing identifying characteristics of individuals or research settings by employing pseudonyms and modifying situations and events.

SUMMARY

In summary, the goal of ethnographers is to describe the experiences of others faithfully within an ethical framework based upon respect for individual autonomy and the treatment of individuals as "ends in themselves, never merely as means" (Cassell, 1980, p. 32). Formal codes and institutional rules provide guidance for research dilemmas, but the crucial imperative to behave morally at all times is the responsibility of each individual investigator. If you embrace a role that provides an opportunity to observe, communicate, and learn from others in a way that is acceptable to them, "It is a *good* role" (Wax, 1971, p. 55, emphasis in original). Maintenance of an ethical relationship with group members depends on several principles:

- Identify personal, cultural, and professional belief systems that may produce biases during the research process. Acknowledge the effects of "culture shock" in an unfamiliar environment.

- Establish a comfortable and productive research role as both insider and outsider to group members.

- Allow subjects to make informed decisions regarding their participation in the research project by providing truthful and specific information. Renegotiate consent as necessary. Specify how the results will be used.

9

ANNOTATED BIBLIOGRAPHY

The following references have been selected to annotate because they are examples of nurse-conducted focused ethnography using participant observation methods. We provide examples from the available literature and not a list of all such studies. Each ethnography is annotated by purpose of the study, including focused and long-term aims, sample/population, and ethnographic methods used by the researcher. Triangulation of methods is identified when present.

Aamodt, A. M. (1979). Social-cultural dimensions of caring in the world of the Papago child and adolescent. In M. Leininger (Ed.), *Transcultural nursing* (pp. 47 56). New York: Masson International Nursing Publications.

The foundation for this paper was the 13 months of ethnographic field-work conducted by the author in the late 1960s. The paper described the world of the children in the Papago reservation in order to contribute to ethnonursing knowledge. Data about the children were collected using participant observation and interviews conducted with the children, their families, and the staff at the school.

Adams, J., Kotanba, J. A., Wardell, D., Sherwood, G., Engebretson, J., & Salmon, L. (1996). An ethnographic assessment of an academic nursing center. *Journal of the American Academy of Nurse Practitioners, 8,* 365-371.

The purpose of this study was to describe and analyze the day-to-day operation of a nurse-practitioner nursing center in a university health science center. Specific questions that directed the research were identified. Using a team approach in data collection (members of a graduate seminar in qualitative research in nursing), the study involved naturalistic observation of routine activities and semistructured interviews with clients and select staff members in the nursing center.

Anderson, N. L. (1996). Decisions about substance abuse among adolescents in juvenile detention. *Image: Journal of Nursing Scholarship, 28*(1), 65-70.

This qualitative study was conducted to discover the perspective of the detained adolescents. The interaction dynamics among young women in juvenile detention were explored. Participant observation helped the investigator learn what it means to live and work behind locked gates. Three methods were used for data collection: group discussion, individual interviews, and participant observation (thus, triangulation of data was performed).

Brink, P. J. (1989). The fattening room among the Annang of Nigeria. *Medical Anthropology, 12,* 131-143.

The purpose of this study was to describe the custom and ceremony of fattening among adolescent girls in Nigeria. Formal and informal interviews were conducted with participants of the process. Only minimal observation was reported, as members of the cultural group considered the events secret. Field notes were substantiated with published accounts of other investigators.

Brink, P. J. (1982). Traditional birth attendants among the Annang of Nigeria. *Social Science and Medicine, 16,* 1883-1892.

This paper compared the practices of rural Annang birth attendants with those of American and Nigerian obstetrical teams and described a proposed training program for Annang traditional birth attendants. Participant observation of birth activities and formal and informal interviews were conducted during 1974-1975 and 1980.

Davis, D. L. (1992). The meaning of menopause in a Newfoundland fishing village. In J. M. Morse (Ed.), *Qualitative health research* (pp. 145-169). Newbury Park, CA: Sage.

The author compared the findings of two research approaches to the meaning of menopause in Grey Rock Harbor, a fishing village on the coast of Newfoundland. Ethnographic methods of participant observation and interviews were found to provide a greater understanding of the meaning of menopause than a quantitative approach.

Dreher, M. C., & Hayes, J. S. (1993). Triangulation in cross-cultural research of child development in Jamaica. *Western Journal of Nursing Research, 15,* 216-229.

This study was conducted for two reasons: to evaluate effects of cannabis consumed during pregnancy by women in Jamaica on their children and to increase understanding about the use of cannabis by Jamaican women. The researchers used both ethnographic field methods (observation and interviews) and standard evaluation tools. Triangulation of data collection and findings were explained in detail.

Evaneshko, V. (1982). Tonawanda Seneca childbearing culture. In M. Kay (Ed.), *Anthropology of human birth* (pp. 395-412). Philadelphia: F. A. Davis.

The study described the childbearing practices of one Native American tribe of New York. Participant observation data were obtained over a period of several years. The investigator lived in a reservation home, participated in group activities, observed childbearing and child-rearing practices, and interviewed residents.

Field, P. A. (1983). An ethnography: Four public health nurses perspectives of nursing. *Journal of Advanced Nursing 8,* 3-12.

Participant observation, formal and informal interviews, client records, and clinic reports were used by the author to obtain thick description of social meanings and cultural motives that made up four nurses' models of nursing. Each nurse's model rested on one underlying philosophical assumption; assumptions varied from seeking a better life to focusing on the problems associated with public health nursing.

Fisher, B. J., & Peterson, C. (1993). She won't be dancing much anyway: A study of surgeons, surgical nurses, and elderly patients. *Qualitative Health Research, 3*, 165-183.

The purpose of this study was to examine ways in which attitudes of surgical personnel toward elderly patients affect their behavior toward patients in the operating room. Methods included 5 months of participant observation in one operating room and a survey questionnaire of 80% of doctors and nurses who worked in the surgical area.

Germain, C. P. (1979). *The cancer unit: An ethnography.* Wakefield, MA: Nursing Resources.

The goal of this study was an ethnographic description of an oncology unit. Specific attention was given to the various roles that nurses play in this subculture. The unit was examined by its functional systems: administration, doctors, nurses, and patients. The researcher assumed primarily the role of observer-as-participant.

Golander, H. (1992). Under the guise of passivity: We can communicate warmth, caring, and respect. In J. M. Morse (Ed.), *Qualitative health research.* Thousand Oaks, CA: Sage.

The purpose of this paper was to reveal the active role that even disabled residents could demonstrate in shaping their everyday lives in a nursing home. The method used was observation alone for 1 year, although the researchers acknowledged verbal interactions with the residents.

Holland, C. K. (1993). An ethnographic study of nursing culture as an exploration for determining the existence of a system of ritual. *Journal of Advanced Nursing, 18,* 1461-1470.

The ritual behaviors within a nursing cultural group were explored. A group of nurses were observed to determine if rituals existed. Participant observation was the ethnographic method of data collection. Insider/outsider issues were discussed.

Horn, B. (1979). Transcultural nursing and child-rearing of the Muckleshoot people. In M. Leininger (Ed.), *Transcultural nursing* (pp. 57-69). New York: Masson International Nursing Publications.

In this paper, the author's purpose was to describe the child-rearing practices among the Muckleshoot, a tribe located in the state of Washington. Interviews and observations of a well-child clinic on the reservation provided the data for the description.

Hutchinson, S. H. (1984). Creating meaning out of horror: How NICU nurses survive and work productively in a stressful environment. *Nursing Outlook, 32*(2), 86-90.

The author used participant observation to understand the culture of a 20-bed newborn intensive care unit in a large hospital and the meaning of events to the nursing staff. Structured interviews were conducted with nurses, as well as informal conversation with nurses on all shifts to clarify observations. The study was conducted across 4 months.

Hyland, L., & Morse, J. M. (1995). Orchestrating comfort: The role of funeral directors. *Death Studies, 19,* 452-474.

Through the use of unstructured in-depth interviews with five funeral directors and nine family members and the participant observation role, the authors were able to describe the behaviors of funeral directors within the context of the specific environment (various locations within the setting).

Jackson, B. S. (1975). An experience in participant observation. *Nursing Outlook, 23,* 552-555.

This study explored the process of adaptation by patients who had emergency colostomies. The author described the challenges she faced while attempting to be a neutral observer in a setting where she was recognized as an "expert." Nine patients were included in this sample.

Kauffman, K. S. (1995). Center as haven: Findings of an urban ethnography. *Nursing Research, 44,* 231-236.

The investigator conducted a 3-year ethnography of a Philadelphia senior center. Data were collected through participant observation, formal interviews, and casual conversations. Primary study participants included members of the center and their friends and relatives.

Kay, M. A. (1977). Health and illness in a Mexican American barrio. In E. H. Spicer (Ed.), *Ethnic medicine in the Southwest* (pp. 99-166). Tucson: University of Arizona Press.

The investigator conducted an ethnographic analysis of a Mexican American barrio to answer the question: "What do we need to know about people in order to tailor health care to them?" Methods included extensive participant observation, formal and informal interviews, and the development of a taxonomy of illnesses common in the community.

Kayser-Jones, J. S. (1981). *Old, alone, and neglected: Care of the aged in the United States and Scotland.* Berkeley: University of California Press.

The purpose of this study was to examine criteria for quality care of the institutionalized aged. A cross-cultural comparison of one long-term care institution in Scotland and one in the United States was conducted. Methods included in-depth participant observation in the two facilities and interviews of 25% of the patients in each institution.

Leininger, M. (1979). The Gadsup of New Guinea and early child-caring behaviors with nursing care implications. In M. Leininger (Ed.), *Transcultural nursing* (pp. 167-185). New York: Masson International Nursing Publications.

The purpose of this research was to study the cultural patterns and values, as well as the health-illness and caring styles of the Gadsup people of New Guinea. The author lived with the Gadsup for about 13 months during the early 1960s. In this chapter, the author focuses on child-rearing patterns.

Lipson, J., Hosseini, M., Kabir, A., Omidian, P., & Edmonston, F. (1995). Health issues among Afghan women in California. *Health Care for Women International, 16,* 279-286.

Ethnographic data related to the difficulties faced by Afghan refugees in the United States were collected for more than 10 years. These data included intensive interviewing, visiting in homes of several families, participating in social occasions, driving individuals to scheduled appointments, and acting as advocates with health or social service providers. Among other findings, the researchers learned that inadequate or misunderstood information contributed to problems in obtaining health care services for many members of the community.

Morse, J. M. (1984). The cultural context of infant feeding in Fiji. *Ecology of Food and Nutrition, 14,* 287-296.

Participant observation in a postnatal unit and postnatal clinic, open-ended interviews with birth attendants and elderly women, and a survey of medical records of infants and siblings were used to describe the cultural beliefs and practices related to infant feeding in Fijian and Fiji-Indian cultures. The study was conducted in the Ba district of the island Viti Levu over a 5-month period. Triangulation of research methods was described.

Morse, J. M. (1989). Cultural variation in behavioral response to parturition: Childbirth in Fiji. *Medical Anthropology, 12,* 35-54.

The purpose of this research was to examine birthing practices in Fiji. Specifically, methods of childbirth to control pain and reduce risk of injury were compared and contrasted, as well as maternal responses to pain. Data were gathered initially by interviews and participant observation in hospitals and villages. These data were then used as a basis for hypothesis development, the continued use of ethnographic methods, and the use of quantitative methods to test research questions. The study was conducted over 6 months. Pain was measured using the Morse Pain Stimulus Scale.

Muecke, M. A. (1992). Mother sold food, daughter sells her body: The cultural continuity of prostitution. *Social Science and Medicine, 35,* 891-901.

The purpose of this article was to present an interpretation of female prostitution in a Buddhist Thai society. The author spent 5 years in northern Thailand gathering participant observation and interview data from 400 urban families and from her participation in activities organized by women's groups. Written materials related to the subject of prostitution were studied to contextualize the place of prostitution in the culture.

Seed, A. (1995). Conducting a longitudinal study: An unsanitized account. *Journal of Advanced Nursing, 21,* 845-852.

The purpose of the research was to describe the experiences of a group of 23 student nurses during their 3-year training program. The purpose of the paper was to present the experiences faced by the researcher during the 3-year study that are not part of the "usual" information written about qualitative investigations.

Thompson, J. (1991). Exploring gender and culture with Khmer refugee women: Reflections on participatory feminist research. *Advances in Nursing Science, 13*(3), 30-48.

The purpose of this year-long study was to explore the adjustment of 16 Khmer refugee women in the United States. The researchers focused specifically on the traditional and cultural values held by the subjects. A secondary aim was to provide support to the women as they made their adjustment through the exploration of their values. Ethnographic interviews were conducted related to women's roles, myths, and dreams. Trauma histories were obtained from some women. A total of 80 hours of participant observation, interviewing, dream analysis, and study of myths were recorded using field notes.

Walker, V. H. (1967). *Nursing and ritualistic practice.* New York: Macmillan.

The purpose of this study was to examine the rituals associated with nursing practice. Rituals included writing nurses' notes, taking vital signs, writing of the shift report, and reporting incidents. Participant observation activities occurred with 171 nursing personnel and 166 junior and senior medical students.

Williams, T. R., & Williams, M. M. (1959). The socialization of the student nurse. *Nursing Research, 8,*18-25.

The purpose of this project was to examine the process of socialization among student nurses. The research was conducted over a 6-year period in five schools of nursing within the United States. Methods of data collection included participant observation, informal interviews, and a survey of written documents to determine the educational philosophies of the selected nursing schools.

Wing, D. M. (1990). A cross-cultural field study of nurses and political strategies. *Western Journal of Nursing Research, 12,* 373-385.

The purpose of this study was to explore the political strategies used by two groups of nurses (United States and Great Britain) to effectively use health care resources. Fifteen nurses were key informants. Several hundred nurses were observed during the 5 months of data collection. The Pfeffer framework provided a model for understanding the politics of health care. The author used analytic induction as the method of analysis. Data collection and analysis occurred simultaneously. New cases were selected based on gaps in theory. When no new discoveries in relation to the theoretical framework were obtained, data collection ceased.

Wolf, Z. R. (1988). *Nurses' work: The sacred and the profane.* Philadelphia: University of Pennsylvania Press.

This ethnography examined nursing rituals involving nurses, patients, and other hospital workers who interacted within a medical unit of a large urban hospital. Data collection occurred over a 12-month period. Methods included participant observation, intensive semistructured interviews, and event analyses.

REFERENCES

Adler, P. A., & Adler, P. (1993). Ethical issues in self-censorship: Ethnographic research on sensitive topics. In C. M. Renzetti & R. M. Lee (Eds.), *Researching sensitive topics* (pp. 249-266). Newbury Park: Sage.

Agar, M. (1973). *Ripping and running: A formal ethnography of urban heroin addicts*. New York: Seminar.

Agar, M. H. (1980). *The professional stranger: An informal introduction to ethnography*. San Diego, CA: Academic Press.

Agar, M. H. (1986). *Speaking of ethnography*. Newbury Park, CA: Sage.

Agar, M. H. (1996). Show it, don't tell it. How to run an ethnography appreciation course. *Practicing Anthropology, 18*(2), 3-5.

Anderson, N. L. (1996). Decisions about substance abuse among adolescents in juvenile detention. *Image: Journal of Nursing Scholarship, 28*(1), 65-70.

Armendariz, A., Saunders, J. M., Poston, S. L., & Valente, S. M. (1997). Exploring a life history of HIV disease and self caring. Alfredo's story. *Journal of the Association of Nurses in AIDS Care, 8*(2), 72-82.

Bartlett, J. (1968). *Bartlett's familiar quotations* (14th ed.). Boston: Little, Brown.

Becker, H. S., & Geer, B. (1984). Participant observation: The analysis of qualitative field data. In R. G. Burgess (Ed.), *Field research: A sourcebook and field manual* (pp. 239-250). London: Allen & Unwin.

Bernard, H. R. (1994). *Research methods in anthropology: Qualitative and quantitative approaches* (2nd ed.). Thousand Oaks, CA: Sage.

Bernard, H. R., & Ryan, G. W. (1998). Text analysis: Qualitative and quantitative methods. In H. R. Bernard (Ed.), *Handbook of methods in cultural anthropology*. Walnut Creek, CA: Altamira.

Bogdan, R., & Biklen, S. K. (1992). *Qualitative research for education: An introduction to theory and method* (2nd ed.). Boston: Allyn & Bacon.

135

Bootzin, R. R., Sechrest, L., Scott, A., & Hannah, M. (1992). Common methodological problems in health services research. *EGAD Quarterly, 1*(3), 101-107.

Borgatti, S. P. (1992). *ANTHROPAC 4.0*. Columbia, SC: Analytic Technologies.

Boyle, J. (1994). Style of ethnography. In J. M. Morse (Ed.), *Critical issues in qualitative research methods* (pp. 159-185). Thousand Oaks, CA: Sage.

Briggs, J. L. (1970). *Never in anger*. Cambridge, MA: Harvard University Press.

Brink, P. J. (1976). *Transcultural nursing: A book of readings*. Englewood Cliffs, NJ: Prentice Hall.

Brink, P. J. (1982). Traditional birth attendants among the Annang of Nigeria. *Social Science and Medicine, 16*, 1883-1892.

Brink, P. J. (1989a). The fattening room among the Annang of Nigeria. *Medical Anthropology, 12*, 131-143.

Brink, P. J. (1989b). Issues in reliability and validity. In J. M. Morse (Ed.), *Qualitative nursing research: A contemporary dialogue* (pp. 151-168). Rockville, MD: Aspen.

Brink, P. J. (1993). Studying African women's secret societies. In C. M. Renzetti & R. M. Lee (Eds.), *Researching sensitive topics* (pp. 235-248). Newbury Park, CA: Sage.

Brink, P. J., & Saunders, J. M. (1976). Culture shock: Theoretical and applied. In P. J. Brink (Ed.), *Transcultural nursing: A book of readings* (pp. 126-138). Englewood Cliffs, NJ: Prentice Hall.

Brink, P. J., & Wood, M. J. (1994). *Basic steps in planning nursing research: From question to proposal* (4th ed.). Boston: Jones & Bartlett.

Burgess, R. G. (1984a). *Field research: A sourcebook and field manual*. London: Allen & Unwin.

Burgess, R. G. (1984b). *In the field: An introduction to field research*. London: Allen & Unwin.

Byerly, E. L. (1969). The nurse researcher as participant-observer in a nursing setting. *Nursing Research, 18*, 230-236.

Carr, G. (1996). Ethnography of an HIV hotel. *Journal of Nurses in AIDS Care, 7*(2), 35-42.

Cassell, J. (1992). Ethical principles for conducting fieldwork. *American Anthropologist, 82*(1), 28-41.

Chagnon, N. A. (1992). *Yanomano* (4th ed.). Fort Worth, TX: Harcourt Brace.

Cohen, M. Z., Knafl, K., & Dzurec, L. C. (1993). Grant writing for qualitative research. *Image: Journal of Nursing Scholarship, 25*(2), 151-156.

Connelly, L. M., Keele, B., Kleinbeck, S., & Schneider, J. (1993). A place to be yourself: Empowerment from the client's perspective. *Image: The Journal of Nursing Scholarship, 25*(4), 297-303.

Cook, L. S., & de Mange, B. P. (1995). Gaining access to Native American cultures by non-native American nursing researchers. *Nursing Forum, 30*(1), 5-9.

Davis, D. L. (1992). The meaning of menopause in a Newfoundland fishing village. In J. M. Morse (Ed.), *Qualitative health research* (pp. 145-169). Newbury Park, CA: Sage.

Delaney, W., & Ames, G. (1993). Integration and exchange in multidisciplinary alcohol research. *Social Science and Medicine, 37*, 5-13.

Denzin, N. (1978). *The research act: A theoretical introduction to sociological methods*. New York: McGraw-Hill.

Diamond, T. (1992). *Making gray gold: Narratives of nursing home care*. Chicago: University of Chicago Press.

Dreher, M. C., & Hayes, J. S. (1993). Triangulation in cross-cultural research of child development in Jamaica. *Western Journal of Nursing Research, 15,* 216-229.

Engebretson, J. (1996). Comparison of nurses and alternate healers. *Image: Journal of Nursing Scholarship, 28,* 95-99.

Estroff, S. E. (1981). *Making it crazy: An ethnography of psychiatric clients in an American community.* Berkeley: University of California Press.

Fetterman, D. M. (1989). *Ethnography step by step.* Newbury Park, CA: Sage.

Field, R. A. (1983). An ethnography: Four public health nurses' perspectives of nursing. *Journal of Advanced Nursing, 8,* 3-12.

Field, P. A. (1989). Doing fieldwork in your own culture. In J. M. Morse (Ed.), *Qualitative nursing research: A contemporary dialogue* (pp. 79-91). Rockville, MD: Aspen.

Fisher, B. J., & Peterson, C. (1993). She won't be dancing much anyway: A study of surgeons, surgical nurses, and elderly patients. *Qualitative Health Research, 3,* 165-183.

Floyd, J. (1993). The use of across-method triangulation in the study of sleep concerns in healthy older adults. *Advances in Nursing Science, 16*(2), 70-80.

Gagliari, B. A. (1991). The family's experience of living with a child with Duchenne muscular dystrophy. *Applied Nursing Research, 4*(4), 159-164.

Gans, H. J. (1984). The participant observer as a human being: Observations on the personal aspects of fieldwork. In R. G. Burgess (Ed.), *Field research: A sourcebook and field manual* (pp. 53-61). London: Allen & Unwin.

Germain, C. P. (1979). *The cancer unit: An ethnography.* Wakefield, MA: Nursing Resources.

Germain, C. (1986). Ethnography: The method.. In P. L. Munhall & C. J. Oiler (Eds.), *Nursing research: A qualitative perspective* (pp. 147-162). Norwalk, CT: Appleton Century Crofts.

Germain, C. (1993). In P. L. Munhall & C. J. Oiler (Eds.), *Nursing research: A qualitative perspective* (2nd ed., pp. 237-268). New York: National League for Nursing Press.

Glaser, B. G., & Strauss, A. L. (1967). *The discovery of grounded theory: Strategies for qualitative research.* Chicago: Aldine.

Golander, H. (1992). Under the guise of passivity: We can communicate warmth, caring, and respect. In J. M. Morse (Ed.), *Qualitative health research.* Newbury Park, CA: Sage.

Gordon, D. F. (1987). Getting close by staying distant: Fieldwork with proselytizing groups. *Qualitative Sociology, 10,* 267-287.

Gross, D. R. (1984). Time allocation: A tool for the study of cultural behavior. *Annual Review of Anthropology, 13,* 519-558.

Hammersley, M., & Arkinson, P. (1983). *Ethnography: Principles in practice.* New York: Tavistock.

Handwerker, W. P., & Borgatti, S. P. (1998). Reasoning with numbers. In H. R. Bernard (Ed.), *Handbook of methods in cultural anthropology.* Walnut Creek, CA: Altamira.

Harris, M. (1928). *The rise of anthropological theory.* New York: Thomas Y. Crowell.

Holland, K. H. (1993). An ethnographic study of nursing culture as an exploration for determining the existence of a system of ritual. *Journal of Advanced Nursing, 18,* 1461-1470.

Hutchinson, S. H. (1984). Creating meaning out of horror: How NICU nurses survive and work productively in a stressful environment. *Nursing Outlook, 32,* 86-90.

Hyland, L., & Morse, J. M. (1995). Orchestrating comfort: The role of funeral directors. *Death Studies, 19,* 453-474.

Hymes, D. (1972). Models of the interaction of language and social life. In J. J. Gumperez & D. Hymes (Eds.), *Directions in sociolinguistics*. New York: Holt, Rinehart & Winston.

Jackson, B. S. (1975). An experience in participant observation. *Nursing Outlook, 23*, 552-555.

Johnson, A. W. (1978). *Quantification in cultural anthropology: An introduction to research design*. Stanford, CA: Stanford University Press.

Johnson, A., & Johnson, O. (1990). Quality and quantity: On the measurement potential of ethnographic fieldnotes. In R. Sanjek (Ed.), *Fieldnotes: The makings of anthropology* (pp. 161-186). Ithaca, NY: Cornell University Press.

Jorgensen, D. L. (1989). *Participant observation: A methodology for human studies*. Newbury Park, CA: Sage.

Kauffman, K. S. (1994). The insider/outsider dilemma: Field experience of a white researcher "getting in" a poor black community. *Nursing Research, 43*, 179-183.

Kauffman, K. S. (1995). Center as haven: Findings of an urban ethnography. *Nursing Research, 44*, 231-236.

Kay, M. A. (1977). Health and illness in a Mexican American barrio. In E. H. Spicer (Ed.), *Ethnic medicine in the Southwest* (pp. 99-166). Tucson: University of Arizona Press.

Khazoyan, C. M., & Anderson, N. L. R. (1994). Latinas' expectations of their partners during childbirth. *Maternal and Child Nursing, 19*, 226-229.

Kleinman, A. (1992). Local worlds of suffering: An interpersonal focus for ethnographies of illness experience. *Qualitative Health Research, 2*, 127-134.

Kleinman, S., & Copp, M. (1993). *Emotions and fieldwork*. Newbury Park, CA: Sage.

Kulig, J. C. (1988). Conception and birth control use: Cambodian refugee women's beliefs and practices. *Journal of Community Health Nursing, 5*(4), 235-246.

Kulig, J. C. (1995). Cambodian refugees' family planning knowledge and use. *Journal of Advanced Nursing, 22*, 150-157.

Lamb, G. S., & Huttlinger, K. (1989). Reflexivity in nursing research. *Western Journal of Nursing Research, 11*, 765-772.

Landy, D. (1977). *Culture, disease, and healing: Studies in medical anthropology*. New York: Macmillan.

LeCompte, M. D., & Goetz, J. P. (1982). Problems of reliability and validity in ethnographic research. *Review of Educational Research, 52*(1), 31-60.

Lee, R., & Renzetti, C. (1993). The problem of researching sensitive topics: An overview and introduction. In C. M. Renzetti & R. M. Lee (Eds.), *Researching sensitive topics* (pp. 3-13). Newbury Park, CA: Sage.

Leininger, M. (1970). *Nursing and anthropology: Two worlds to blend*. New York: John Wiley.

Leininger, M. M. (1985). *Qualitative research methods in nursing*. Orlando, FL: Grune & Stratton.

Levi-Strauss, C. (1963). *Structural anthropology*. New York: Basic Books.

Lincoln, Y. S., & Guba, E. G. (1985). *Naturalistic inquiry*. Beverly Hills, CA: Sage.

Lipson, J. G. (1984). Combining researcher, clinical and personal roles: Enrichment or confusion? *Human Organization, 43*, 348-352.

Lipson, J. G. (1989). The use of self in ethnographic research. In J. M. Morse (Ed.), *Qualitative nursing research: A contemporary dialogue* (pp. 61-75). Rockville, MD: Aspen.

Lipson, J. B. (1994). Ethical issues in ethnography. In J. M. Morse (Ed.), *Critical issues in qualitative research methods*. Thousand Oaks, CA: Sage.

Lipson, J. G., Hosseini, T., Kabir, S., Omidian, P. A., & Edmonston, F. (1995). Health issues among Afghan women in California. *Health Care for Women International, 16,* 279-286.

Lipson, J. G., & Meleis, A. I. (1989). Methodological issues in research with immigrants. *Medical Anthropology, 12,* 103-115.

Lipson, J. G., & Omidian, P. A. (1997). Afghan refugee issues in the U.S. social environment. *Western Journal of Nursing Research, 19,* 110-126.

Lofland, J. (1971). *Analyzing social settings: A guide to qualitative observation and analysis.* Belmont, CA: Wadsworth.

Lowenberg, J. S. (1993). Interpretive research methodology: Broadening the dialogue. *Advances in Nursing Science, 16*(2), 57-69.

MacDonald, H. (1996). Mastering uncertainty: Mothering the child with asthma. *Pediatric Nursing 22*(1), 55-59.

Magilvy, J. K., McMahon, M., Backman, M., Roark, S., & Evenson, C. (1987). The health of teenagers: a focused ethnography. *Public Health Nursing 4*(1), 35-42.

Malinowski, B. (1922). *Argonauts of the western Pacific.* New York: Dutton.

Marcus, G., & Fischer, M. (1986). *Anthropology as cultural critique.* Chicago: University of Chicago Press.

Mayo, K. (1992). Physical activity practices among American black working women. *Qualitative Health Research 2,* 318-333.

McCall, G. J., & Simmons, J. L. (Eds.). (1969). *Issues in participant observation: A text and reader.* Reading, MA: Addison-Wesley.

McGarrahan, P. (1994). *Transcending AIDS: Nurses and HIV patients in New York City.* Philadelphia: University of Pennsylvania Press.

Mead, M. (1968). *Coming of age in Samoa: A psychological study of primitive youth for Western civilization.* New York: Morrow.

Miles, M. B., & Huberman, A. M. (1994). *An expanded sourcebook: Qualitative data analysis.* Thousand Oaks, CA: Sage.

Morse, J. M. (1984). The cultural context of infant feeding in Fiji. *Ecology of Food and Nutrition, 14,* 287-296.

Morse, J. M. (1987). Qualitative nursing research: a free-for-all? In J. M. Morse (Ed.), *Qualitative nursing research: A contemporary dialogue* (pp. 14-22). Newbury Park, CA: Sage.

Morse, J. M. (1989). Strategies for sampling. In J. M. Morse (Ed.), *Qualitative nursing research: A contemporary dialogue* (pp. 117-131). Rockville, MD: Aspen.

Morse, J. M. (1991). Editorial: Evaluation of qualitative proposals. *Qualitative Health Research, 1,* 147-151.

Morse, J. M., & Field, P. A. (1995). *Qualitative research methods for health professionals* (2nd ed.). Thousand Oaks, CA: Sage.

Muecke, M. A. (1992). Nursing research with refugees. *Western Journal of Nursing Research, 14,* 703-770.

Muecke, M. A. (1994). On the evaluation of ethnographies. In J. M. Morse (Ed.), *Critical issues in qualitative research methods* (pp. 187-209). Thousand Oaks, CA: Sage.

Munhall, P. L. (1988). Ethical considerations in qualitative research. *Western Journal of Nursing Research, 10,* 150-162.

Osborne, O. H. (1969). Anthropology and nursing: Some common traditions and interests. *Nursing Research, 18,* 251-255.

Pelto, P. J., & Pelto, G. H. (1978). *Anthropological research: The structure of inquiry* (2nd ed.). Cambridge, UK: Cambridge University Press.

Powdermaker, H. (1966). *Stranger and friend: The way of an anthropologist.* Toronto: McLeod.

Preston, R. M. (1997). Ethnography: Studying the fate of health promotion in coronary families. *Journal of Advanced Nursing 25,* 554-561.

Proctor, A., Morse, J. M., & Khnosari, E. S. (1996). Sounds of comfort in the trauma center: How nurses talk to patients in pain. *Social Science and Medicine, 42,* 1669-1680.

Ragucci, A. T. (1972). The ethnographic approach and nursing research. *Nursing Research, 21,* 485-490.

Rhodes, L. A. (1991). *Emptying beds: The work of an emergency psychiatric unit.* Berkeley: University of California Press.

Romney, A. K., Weller, S. C., & Batchelder, W. H. (1986). Culture as consensus. *American Anthropologist 88,* 313-338.

Roper, J. M., & Anderson, N. L. (1991). The influence of interactional variables on violence on an acute inpatient psychiatric ward: Part I. *Archives of Psychiatric Nursing, 4,* 209-215.

Roper, J. M., & Shapira, J. (1999). *Nurse caregiver feelings about agitation in Alzheimer's disease.* Paper submitted for publication.

Rosenhan, D. L. (1973). On being sane in insane places. *Science, 179,* 250-258.

Rubel, A. J. (1966). *Across the tracks: Mexican-Americans in a Texas city.* Austin: University of Texas Press.

Salyer, J., & Stuart, B. J. (1985). Nurse-patient interaction in the intensive care unit. *Heart and Lung, 14*(1), 20-24.

Sandelowski, M., Davis, D. H., & Harris, B. G. (1989). Artful design: Writing the proposal for research in the naturalistic paradigm. *Research in Nursing and Health, 12,* 77-84.

Sanjek, R. (1990). *Fieldnotes: The makings of anthropology.* Ithaca, NY: Cornell University Press.

Saunders, J. M., & Valente, S. M. (1992). Nursing research and vulnerable populations. Editors of symposium: Research issues with vulnerable populations. *Western Journal of Nursing Research, 14,* 700-702.

Schatzman, L., & Strauss, A. L. (1973). *Field research: Strategies for a natural sociology.* Englewood Cliffs, NJ: Prentice Hall.

Scheper-Hughes, N. (1979). *Saints, scholars and schizophrenics: Mental illness in rural Ireland.* Berkeley: University of California Press.

Schwartz, M. S., & Schwartz, C. G. (1955). Problems in participant observation. *American Journal of Sociology, 60,* 343-353.

Scotch, N. A. (1963). Medical anthropology. *Biennial Review of Anthropology, 3,* 30-68.

Seed, A. (1995). Conducting a longitudinal study: An unsanitized account. *Journal of Advanced Nursing, 21,* 845-852.

Shaffir, W. B., & Stebbins, R. A. (1991). *Experiencing fieldwork: An inside view of qualitative research.* Newbury Park, CA: Sage.

Shapira, J. (1997, March). *Experiences of psychiatric patients in an evaluation and admissions department: A question of stigma.* Paper presented to the Society for Applied Anthropology, Seattle, WA.

Sherwin, J. S. (1969). *A word index to Walden, with textual notes.* Hartford: Emerson Society.

Silverman, D. (1993). *Interpreting qualitative data: Methods for analyzing talk, text and interaction.* Newbury Park, CA: Sage.

Spradley, J. P. (1970). *You owe yourself a drunk: An ethnography of urban nomads.* Boston: Little, Brown.

Spradley, J. P. (1979). *The ethnographic interview.* Toronto, Canada: Holt, Rinehart and Winston.

Spradley, J. P. (1980). *Participant observation.* Fort Worth, TX: Harcourt Brace Jovanovich.

Spradley, J. P., & McCurdy, D. W. (1972). *The cultural experience: Ethnography in complex society.* Chicago: Science Research Associates.

Stocking, G. W. (1983). *Observers observed: Essays on ethnographic fieldwork.* Madison: University of Wisconsin Press.

Strauss, A. (1987). *Qualitative analysis for social scientists.* Cambridge, UK: Cambridge University Press.

Strauss, A., & Corbin, J. (1990). *Basics of qualitative research: Grounded theory procedures and techniques.* Newbury Park, CA: Sage.

Street, A. F. (1992). *Inside nursing: A critical ethnography of clinical nursing practice.* Albany: State University of New York.

Tripp-Reimer, T., Brink, P., & Saunders, J. (1984). Cultural assessment: Content and process. *Nursing Outlook, 32,* 78-82.

Turner, V. (1967). *The forest of symbols: Aspects of Ndembu ritual.* Ithaca, NY: Cornell University Press.

Wax, R. H. (1971). *Doing fieldwork: Warnings and advice.* Chicago: University of Chicago Press.

Weitzman, E., & Miles, M. (1994). *Computer programs for qualitative data analysis.* Thousand Oaks, CA: Sage.

Weller, S. C. (1987). Shared knowledge, intracultural variation, and knowledge aggregation. *American Behavioral Scientist, 31,* 178-193.

Wellin, E. (1978). Theoretical orientations in medical anthropology: Conceptual, organizational, and educational priorities. *Social Science and Medicine, 5,* 15-36.

Werner, O., & Schoepfle, G. M. (1987). *Systematic fieldwork: Foundations of ethnography and interviewing.* Newbury Park, CA: Sage.

Whiting, B., & Whiting, J. (1973). Methods for observing and recording behavior. In R. Naroll & R. Cohen (Eds.), *A handbook of method in cultural anthropology* (pp. 282-315). New York: Columbia University Press.

Whyte, W. F. (1955). *Street corner society: The social structure of an Italian slum* (2nd ed.). Chicago: University of Chicago Press.

Wilson, H. (1989). The craft of qualitative analysis. In H. Wilson (Ed.), *Research in nursing* (2nd ed., pp.452-499). Redwood City, CO: Addison-Wesley.

Wing, D. M. (1990). A cross-cultural field study of nurses and political strategies. *Western Journal of Nursing Research, 12,* 373-385.

Wolcott, H. F. (1990). *Writing up qualitative research.* Newbury Park, CA: Sage.

AUTHOR INDEX

Aamodt, A. M., 125
Adams, J., 126
Adler, P., 122
Adler, P. A., 122
Agar, M., 122
Agar, M. H., 2, 4, 11, 65, 68, 69, 71, 74, 75, 78, 79, 80, 84, 85
Ames, G., 92
Anderson, N. I., R., 22, 23, 72, 102, 126
Armendariz, A., 122
Atkinson, P., 116

Backman, M., 23, 24, 30, 92, 95
Bartlett, J., 29, 39, 55, 113
Becker, H. S., 13, 93
Bernard, H. R., 2, 72, 81, 82, 104
Biklen, S. K., 94
Bogdan, R., 94
Bootzin, R. R., 50
Borgatti, S. P., 105, 106, 107
Boyle, J., 4
Briggs, J. L., 67, 115
Brink, P. J., 7, 8, 9, 17, 29, 30, 31, 40, 43, 67, 78, 79, 83, 114, 116, 122, 126

Burgess, R. G., 12, 17, 19, 21, 40, 43, 50, 61, 91, 92, 93, 120, 122
Byerly, E. I., 17, 117, 118

Carr, G., 8-9, 14, 35
Cassell, J., 11, 120, 123
Chagnon, N. A., 3, 4
Cohen, M. Z., 40, 43, 48, 50
Connelly, L. M., 92
Cook, L. S., 23, 34, 56, 57
Copp, M., 114
Corbin, J., 42, 85, 94

Davis, D. H., 40, 43, 49
Davis, D. L., 6, 127
de Mange, B. P., 23, 34, 56, 57
Delaney, W., 92
Densin, N., 24
Diamond, T., 21
Dreher, M. C., 12, 22, 24, 30, 127
Dzurec, L. C., 40, 43, 48, 50

Edmonston, F., 8, 130

143

Engebretson, J., 24, 92, 126
Estroff, S., 6
Estroff, S. E., 14, 15
Evaneshko, V., 127
Evenson, C., 23, 24, 30, 92, 95

Fetterman, D. M., 3, 40, 65, 68, 74, 77, 78, 88, 92, 108
Field, P. A., 7, 15, 24, 26, 40, 92, 108, 110, 114, 119, 127
Fischer, M., 115
Fisher, B. J., 14, 128
Floyd, J., 92

Gagliari, B. A., 14
Gans, H. J., 15, 21
Geer, B., 13, 93
Germain, C., 9, 81, 82, 118
Germain, C. P., 9, 13, 16, 19, 57, 63, 128
Glaser, B. G., 78
Goetz, J. P., 82, 83
Golander, H., 42, 128
Gross, D. R., 81
Guba, E. G., 94

Hammersley, M., 116
Handwerker, W. P., 105, 106, 107
Hannah, M., 50
Harris, B. G., 40, 43, 49
Hayes, J. S., 12, 22, 24, 30, 127
Holland, C. K., 128
Holland, K. H., 92
Horn, B., 128
Hosseini, T., 8, 130
Huberman, A. M., 92, 94, 98, 99, 101, 104
Hutchinson, S., 9
Hutchinson, S. H., 129
Huttlinger, K., 115
Hyland, L., 57, 129
Hymes, D., 71

Jackson, B. S., 119, 129
Johnson, A., 72, 85
Johnson, O., 72, 85
Jorgensen, D. L., 83, 102

Kabir, S., 8, 130
Kauffman, K. S., 8, 14, 118, 129

Kay, M., 5-6, 127, 130
Kayser-Jones, J. S., 130
Keele, B., 92
Khazoyan, C. M., 22, 23
Khnosari, F. S., 88
Kleinbeck, S., 92
Kleinman, A., 7
Kleinman, S., 114
Knafl, K., 40, 43, 48, 50
Kotanba, J. A., 126
Kulig, J. C., 15, 22, 92

Lamb, G. S., 115
Landy, D., 5
LeCompte, M. D., 82, 83
Lee, R., 121
Leininger, M. M., 4, 7, 8, 9, 40, 125, 128, 130
Lévi-Strauss, C., 4
Lincoln, Y. S., 94
Lipson, J. B., 120, 121
Lipson, J. G., 8, 15, 22, 115, 118, 119, 121, 130
Lofland, J., 66, 70, 74, 77, 84, 85, 94
Lowenberg, J. S., 11, 12

MacDonald, H., 22, 92
Magilvy, J. K., 23, 24, 30, 92, 95
Malinowski, B., 1, 2-3, 3
Marcus, G., 115
Mayo, K., 35
McCall, G. J., 117
McCurdy, D. W., 3
McGarrahan, P., 79
McMahon, M., 23, 24, 30, 92, 95
Mead, M., 3
Meleis, A. I., 121
Miles, M. B., 92, 94, 98, 99, 101, 104
Morse, J. M., 7, 8, 12, 13, 15, 22, 24, 40, 44, 57, 61, 78, 79, 80, 88, 92, 95, 108, 110, 114, 127, 128, 129, 131
Muecke, M. A., 7, 15, 22, 131
Munhall, P. L., 121

Omidian, P. A., 8, 130
Osborne, O. H., 9

Pelto, G. H., 4, 68, 73
Pelto, P. J., 4, 68, 73

Peterson, C., 14, 128
Poston, S. L., 122
Powdermaker, H., 117
Preston, R. M., 57
Proctor, A., 88

Ragucci, A. T., 12
Renzetti, C., 121
Rhodes, L. A., 69
Rivers, W. H. R., 2
Roark, S., 23, 24, 30, 92, 95
Romney, A. K., 106
Roper, J. M., 25, 30, 31, 32, 33, 44, 75,
    80, 95, 102
Rosenhan, D. I., 20
Rubel, A., 5-6
Ryan, G. W., 104

Salmon, I., 126
Salyer, J., 21
Sandelowski, M., 40, 43, 49
Sanjek, R., 109
Saunders, J. M., 8, 67, 116, 119, 121,
    122
Schatzman, L., 4
Scheper-Hughes, N., 122
Schneider, J., 92
Schoepfle, G. M., 4, 7, 65, 77, 85, 114,
    117
Schwartz, C. G., 17, 20
Schwartz, M. S., 17, 20
Scotch, N. A., 5
Scott, A., 50
Sechrest, L., 50
Seed, A., 18, 117, 118, 131
Shaffir, W. B., 116
Shapira, J., 25, 30, 31, 32, 44, 75, 80,
    107

Sherwin, J. S., 65
Sherwood, G., 126
Silverman, D., 24
Simmons, J. L., 117
Snadelowski, M., 40
Spicer, E. H., 130
Spradley, J. P., 3, 13, 22, 70
Stebbins, R. A., 116
Stocking, G. W., 2
Strauss, A. L., 4, 42, 78, 85, 94
Street, A. F., 9, 12, 19, 20, 26, 27, 57, 63
Stuart, B. J., 21

Thompson, J., 132
Tripp-Reimer, T., 8
Turner, V., 3, 4

Valente, S. M., 121, 122

Walker, V. H., 132
Wardell, D., 126
Wax, R. H., 67, 123
Weitzman, E., 104
Weller, S. C., 106
Wellin, E., 5
Werner, O., 4, 7, 65, 77, 85, 114, 117
Whiting, B., 71
Whiting, J., 71
Whyte, W. F., 3
Williams, M. M., 132
Williams, T. R., 132
Wilson, H., 25
Wing, D. M., 17, 92, 132
Wolcott, H. F., 108, 109
Wolf, Z. R., 133
Wood, M. J., 29, 30, 31, 40, 43, 78, 79,
    83

SUBJECT INDEX

Access, 55-56, 64
    contact process, 61-63
    institutional review board processes,
        56-58
    protection of human subjects, 58-59
    qualitative issues, 59-60
    research approval, 60-61
    scientific merit review, 59
    See also Sampling
Anthropology, viii, 2-3, 12

Behavior patterns. *See* Human behavior
    patterns
Behavioral/materialistic perspective, 3
Bias, 12, 16-17, 16 (table), 70, 114-116

Coding/descriptive labels, 94-98, 96-97
    (table)
Cognitive perspective, 3
Community, 1, 2-3
    holistic ethnography, 3-4
    medical ethnography and, 5-6
Computer technologies:
    consensus analysis, 106-107
    data quantification, 105-107

descriptive statistics, 106
    inferential data analysis, 107
    text analysis, 103 (table), 104-105
Contextual information, 3-4, 6
Culture, 2-5
    behavioral/materialistic perspective, 3
    cognitive perspective, 3
    contextual information, 3-4, 6
    focused ethnography and, 7-9
    health behaviors, 5-6

Data analysis, 47-48, 51, 91-92, 111-112
    coding/descriptive labels, 94-98, 96-97
        (table)
    computer technologies, 104 (table),
        104-107
    constructs/theories, 100-101,
        100 (table)
    inductive process, 13, 93
    memoing, 101-102
    outliers, 99
    principles of, 92-94
    process/procedure, 102-104
    sorting into sets, 96 (table), 98-99
    See also Computer technologies
Data collection, 12, 13, 27, 52

bias, 16-17, 16 (table)
   quantitative measures, 24-25
   reliability, 83
   validation, 15-16, 16 (table), 28, 83
   See also Field notes
Documents, 1-2, 23, 28, 81-82

Emic perspective, 4, 9, 70
Ethics, 113-114, 123
   biases, 114-116
   informed consent, 120-122
   insider/outsider role, 116-120
   professional integrity, 118-120
Ethnography, viii, 1-2, 4-5, 11-12
   culture and, 3-4
   emic/etic perspective, 4, 6, 9, 70
   focused, 7-9
   historical characteristics of, 2-3
   holistic perspective, 3-4, 6
   inductive process of, 13, 93
   nursing practice and, 26-27
   participant observation in, 1-2, 4,
      13-21
   qualitative methods, 11-12, 12 (table)
   reflexive nature of, 4, 26
   See also Medical ethnography;
      Research; Research processes
Etic perspective, 4, 6, 9, 70

Field notes, viii, 2, 84
   complete, 85
   equipment for, 87-88
   importance of, 86-87
   partial, 84-85
   systematic collection, 86
   See also Documentation
Focused ethnography, 7-9
   health beliefs/practices, 7-8
   nursing as cultural system, 9
   subcultural groups, 8-9

Gatekeepers, 34-36
Grounded theory, 11, 12 (table), 13

Health behavior, 5-6
   focused ethnography and, 7-9
Holistic perspective, 3-4

Human behavior patterns, 2-3, 4
   focused ethnography, 7-9
   health and community, 5-6

Inductive process, 13, 93
Informants, 76-78
Information:
   contextual, 3-4, 6
   health care and, 8
   supplementary sources, 81-82
   See also Documentation
Informed consent, 120-122
Insider/outsider role, 116-120
Institutional review boards (IRBs),
   39-40
   processes of, 56-58
   protection of human subjects, 58-59
   qualitative issues, 59-60
   research approval, 60-61
   scientific merit review, 59
Interviewing, 1, 2, 22-23, 28, 73, 76
   formal, 75-76
   group, 73-74
   informal, 74-75

Lifeways, 4

Macroethnography, 7
Medical ethnography, 5-6
   focused inquiry, 7-9
   See also Research
Memoing, 101-102
Miniethnography, 7

Nursing practice:
   cultural systems and, 9
   ethnography and, 26-27
   observation in, 25-26

Observation:
   descriptive, 70, 72
   focused/systematic, 70-71
   genres of, 71
   selective, 71
   speech behavior patterns, 71-72
   See also Participant observation
Outliers, 99

Paper writing, 108-111
Participant observation, 1-2, 4, 13, 27
  dimensions of, 13-17, 16 (table), 28
  exploratory, 66-69
  field notes and, 86-87
  insider/outsider role, 116-120
  levels of, 17-18, 27
  nursing practice and, 25-26
  observer only, 20-21
  bserver-as-participant, 19
  participant only, 21
  participant-as-observer, 18-19
  process of, 70-72
Phenomenology, 11, 12 (table), 13
Proposal, preparation for:
  gatekeeper contact, 34-36
  knowledge level assessment, 31-34
  research question identification,
    29-31
  time/money issues, 36-38
Proposal writing, 39-40, 53
  budgeting, 48-49
  content, 40-41, 41 (table)
  data analysis, 47-48, 51
  ethnographic research and, 49-50
  language in, 48
  letters of support, 49
  literature citations, 43-44, 50
  methodological problems, 50-52
  methodology, 45-47
  significance of study, 44-45, 52
  study aims/hypotheses, 41-43, 49

Qualitative methods, 11-12, 12 (table)
Quantitative measures, 24-25

Records. See Documentation
Reflexivity, 4, 26
Research, 2
  data collection, 12, 13, 15-17, 16
    (table), 27
  documents, 1-2, 23, 28
  focused ethnography, 7-9
  interviews, 22-23, 28
  investigator influence, 12, 70
  participant observation, 13-21
  qualitative framework, 11-12,
    12 (table)

quantitative measures, 24-25
triangulation, 24-25, 28, 51, 83
  See also Access; Proposal, preparation
    for; Proposal writing
Research processes, 65-66, 89
  conclusion, 88-89
  exploratory participant observation,
    66-69
  field notes, 84-88
  gaining entry, 66-68
  information, supplementary sources,
    81-82
  informed consent, 120-122
  interviewing, 73-76
  participant observation, 70-72
  reliability, 83
  sampling, 76-81
  survey, general, 68-69
  validity, 82-83
  writing the paper, 108-111

Sampling:
  events, 80-81
  judgmental/purposeful/theoretical
    sample, 78-79
  key informants, 76-78
  nominated/opportunist/snowball
    sample, 78
  random, 79
  solicited samples, 79
  stratified/quota, 79-80
  total populations, 79
Saturation, 14
SPEAKING (Setting, Participants, Ends,
  Act, Key, Instrumentality, Norms,
  Genre), 71-72
Speech behavior patterns, 71-72

Theories/constructs, 100-101, 100 (table)
Triangulation, 24-25, 28, 51, 83

Validation, 15-16, 16 (table), 22, 24, 28
  quota sampling and, 80
  research design, 82-83

Writing. See Paper writing; Proposal
  writing

ABOUT THE AUTHORS

Janice M. Roper, Ph.D., is currently Director of the Nursing Research Program at the Veterans Administration Greater Los Angeles Healthcare System (VAGLAHS). In this role, she provides consultation, supervision, mentoring, and the coordination of nursing research as well as the conduct of research. She is currently an Assistant Clinical Professor at UCLA. As part of her promotion of nursing research, she teaches classes on research and on qualitative methodology. Her research focuses primarily on nursing issues related to chronic illness, using both quantitative and qualitative methodologies. Her master's thesis and doctoral dissertation used qualitative methodologies. The latter was an ethnography on the use of physical restraints in a psychiatric inpatient setting. She received her doctorate in anthropology from the University of California (UCLA), her master's from UCLA, and her baccalaureate from California State University, Los Angeles. She has published in refereed journals and has presented her research findings at national conferences. She is a reviewer for the *Western Journal of Nursing Research* and is a board member and reviewer for the *Journal of Transcultural Nursing*.

Jill Shapira, an adult nurse practitioner, has clinical practices at both the UCLA Alzheimer's Disease Center and the Veterans Administration Greater Los Angeles Healthcare System. She assists patients with dementia and their families to manage agitated behaviors and other projects and publications she utilizes a qualitative perspective when describing the impact of dementia on individuals. She is also Assistant Clinical Professor at the UCLA School of Nursing. She received her master's and baccalaureate degrees in nursing from UCLA, where she is currently completing fieldwork for a Ph.D. in medical anthropology. Her ethnography explores the world of nurses in one surgical intensive care unit as they interact with patients; how nurses move between and within their individual and nursing subcultures when caring for patients is the focus of study. Through these clinical and research activities she has learned to appreciate and privilege the experiences patients and study participants share with her.